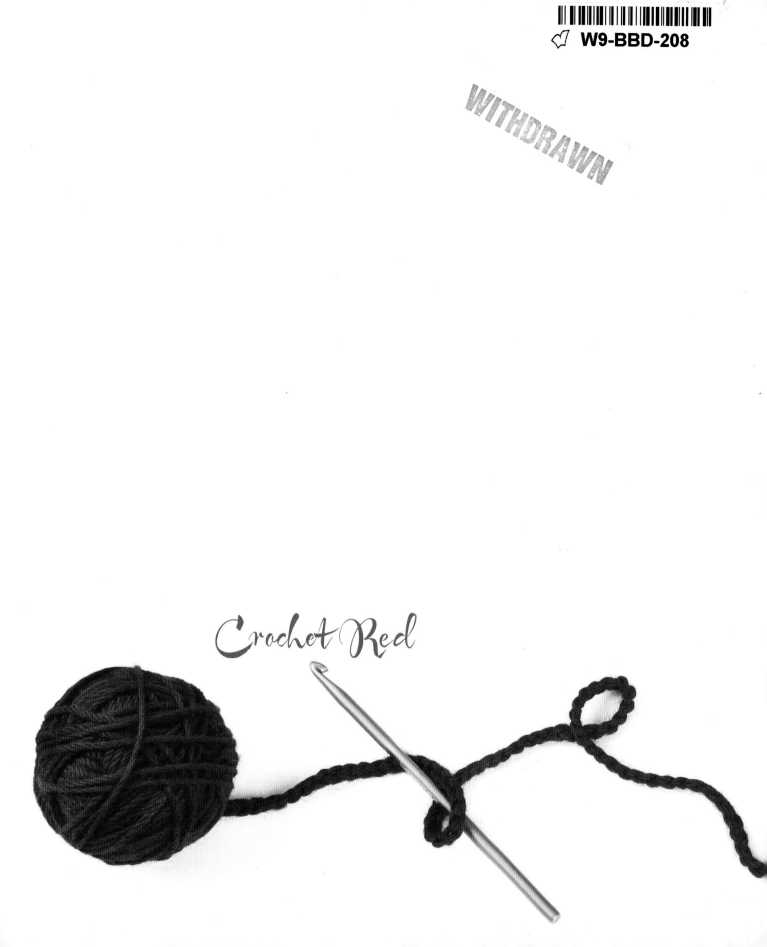

Crochet Red

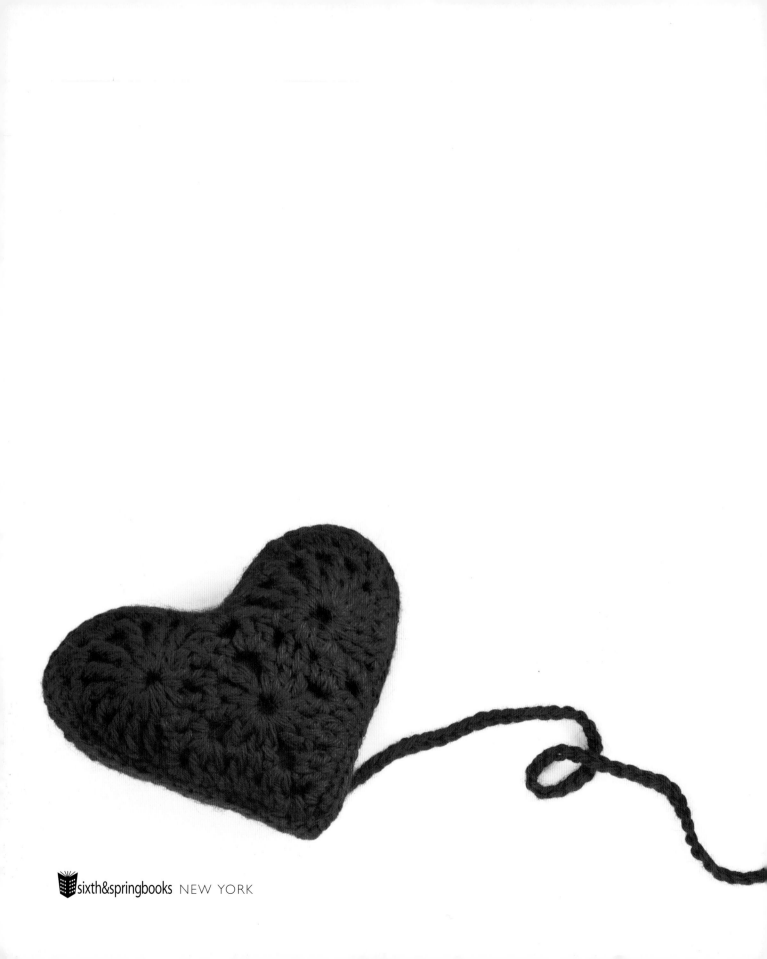

sixth&springbooks NEW YORK

Crochet Red

CROCHETING FOR WOMEN'S HEART HEALTH

LAURA ZANDER

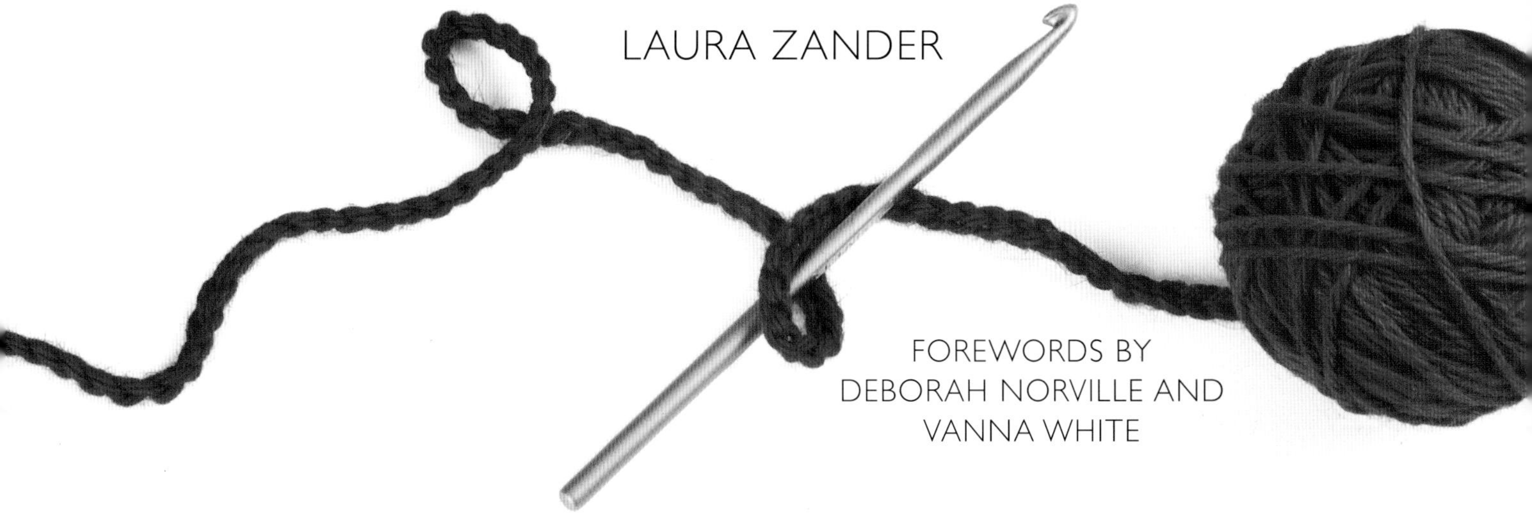

FOREWORDS BY
DEBORAH NORVILLE AND
VANNA WHITE

♥ DEDICATION

This book is dedicated to the hundreds of women who shared their stories of heart disease over the past two years. Thank you for being so honest and open. Keep it up—you are making a difference!

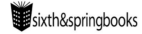

sixth&springbooks

161 Avenue of the Americas, New York, NY 10013

sixthandspringbooks.com

Editorial Director
JOY AQUILINO

Developmental Editor
LISA SILVERMAN

Art Director
DIANE LAMPHRON

Yarn Editor
JOANNA RADOW

Editorial/Art Assistant
JOHANNA LEVY

Page Designer
ARETA BUK

Instructions Editors
ROBYN CHACHULA
K. J. HAY
KIM KOTARY
SHIRI MOR
STEPHANIE MRSE
AMY POLCYN
LORI STEINBERG
MARY BETH TEMPLE
BARBARA VAN ELSEN

Technical Illustrations
LORETTA DACHMAN
ANDREA GRACIARENA
ULI MUNCH

Fashion Stylist
KHALIAH JONES

Model Photography
ROSE CALLAHAN

Still Photography
MARCUS TULLIS

Vice President
TRISHA MALCOLM

Publisher
CARRIE KILMER

Production Manager
DAVID JOINNIDES

President
ART JOINNIDES

Chairman
JAY STEIN

Library of Congress Cataloging-in-Publication Data

Zander, Laura.
 Crochet red : crocheting for women's heart health / Laura Zander.
     pages cm
ISBN 978-1-936096-61-9 (paperback)
1. Crocheting—Patterns. 2. Heart diseases in women—Prevention. I. Title.
TT825.Z35 2014
746.43'4—dc23
                              2013027656

Manufactured in China

1 3 5 7 9 10 8 6 4 2

First Edition

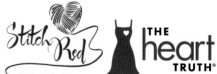

The Heart Truth®, its logo and The Red Dress are registered trademarks of HHS.

Participation by Jimmy Beans Wool does not imply endorsement by HHA/NIH/NHLBI.

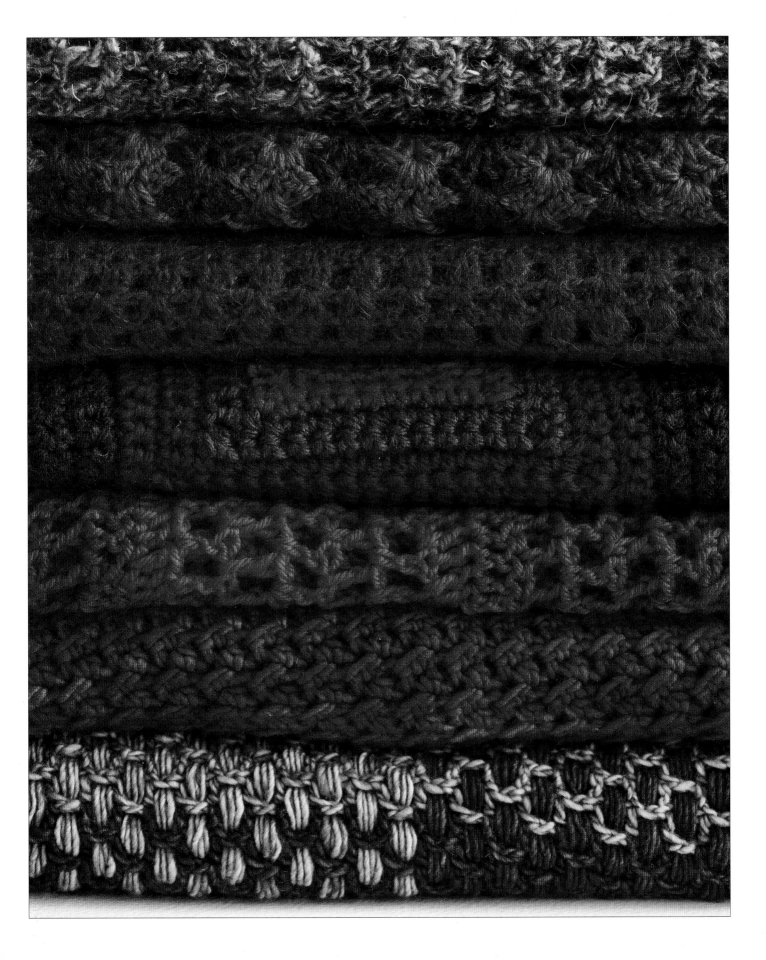

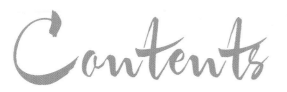

Contents

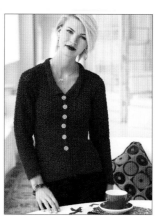

PEPLUM JACKET
page 16
❤ *Kathy Merrick*

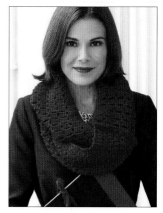

BOBBLE & CHECK COWL
page 22
❤ *Norah Gaughan*

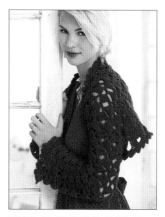

TILTING BLOCKS SHRUG
page 36
❤ *Deborah Norville/*
Rae Blackledge

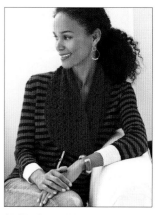

SLOUCHY COWL
page 39
❤ *Edie Eckman*

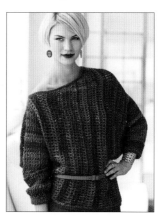

ASYMMETRICAL SWEATER
page 57
❤ *Jenny King*

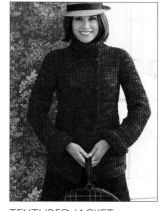

TEXTURED JACKET
page 60
❤ *Melissa Leapman*

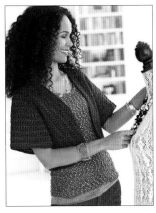

WOVEN CARDIGAN
page 24
♥ *Cornelia Tuttle Hamilton*

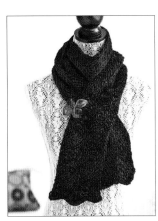

TUNISIAN CHEVRON
SCARF
page 28
♥ *Sharon H. Silverman*

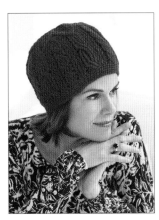

PETAL CABLED HAT
page 31
♥ *Linda Permann*

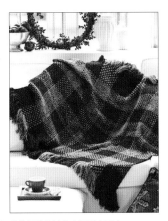

GINGHAM AFGHAN
page 34
♥ *Tanis Galik*

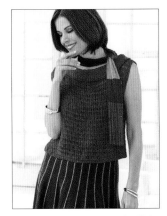

VINTAGE TUNISIAN SHELL
page 42
♥ *Rohn Strong*

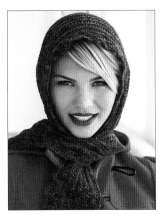

HOODED SCARF
page 45
♥ *Drew Emborsky*

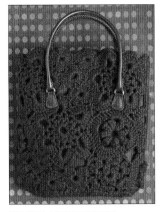

MIXED MOTIF TOTE
page 48
♥ *Erika Knight*

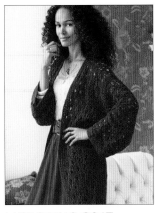

LACE SWING COAT
page 51
♥ *Charles Voth*

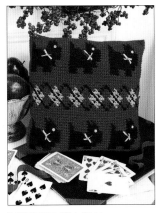

SCOTTIE PILLOW
page 64
♥ *Debbie Bliss/Kathy Merrick*

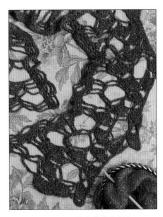

FLOWER LACE SCARF
page 66
♥ *Iris Schreier*

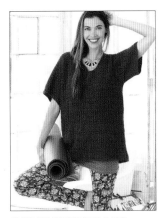

EYELET-STRIPE TUNIC
page 69
♥ *Marie Wallin*

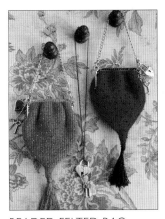

BEADED FELTED BAG
page 73
♥ *Nora Bellows*

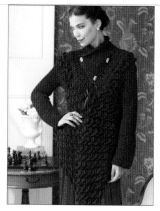

HEART-SHAPED COAT
page 76
❤ *Nicky Epstein*

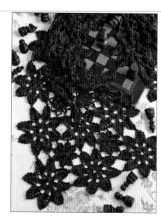

FLORAL MOTIF WRAP
page 81
❤ *Dora Ohrenstein*

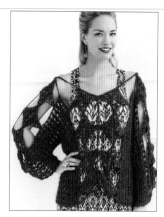

OVERSIZED LACY PULLOVER
page 85
❤ *Deborah Newton*

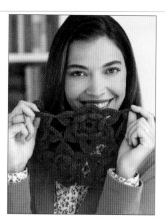

FLOWER GARLAND COWL
page 89
❤ *Robyn Chachula*

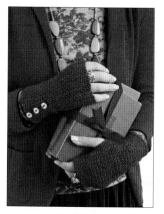

THREE-BUTTON MITTS
page 92
❤ *Kit Hutchin*

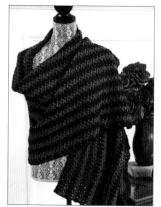

REVERSIBLE WRAP
page 94
❤ *Mary Beth Temple*

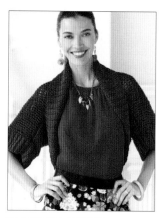

TUNISIAN SHRUG
page 97
❤ *Kristin Omdahl*

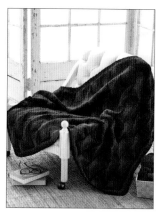

MITERED BRICK THROW
page 102
❤ *Vanna White*

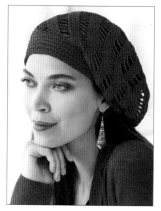

VORTEX SLOUCHY HAT
page 106
❤ *Jill Wright*

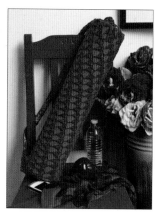

YOGA BAG
page 109
❤ *Vickie Howell*

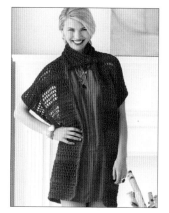

MOCK NECK VEST
page 112
❤ *The Double Stitch Twins*

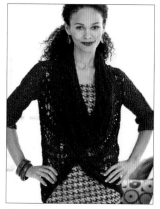

SWEATER WITH COWL
page 116
❤ *Marly Bird*

♥ A MESSAGE FROM THE HEART TRUTH

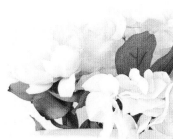

The National Heart, Lung, and Blood Institute's *The Heart Truth*® campaign is proud to have Jimmy Beans Wool and its inspiring campaign Stitch Red, which raises awareness of women's heart disease, as a partner. Our programs share a common goal: to educate women about the risk factors for heart disease and encourage them to take action to protect their heart health.

Stitch Red's mission parallels that of *The Heart Truth*: to give women a personal and urgent wake-up call about their number-one killer—heart disease. *The Heart Truth*, along with its partners, empowers women to make a commitment to managing their potential risk for heart disease. Although a woman's risk increases between the ages of forty and sixty, heart disease can affect women of any age—so it's never too soon or too late to take action for a healthy heart.

Our hope is that you'll be inspired to share the *Heart Truth*® message with friends, family, and fellow crafters, so they become motivated to start making healthy changes in their daily lives. Help each other take the first steps toward a healthy diet: not smoking, getting regular physical activity, and maintaining a healthy weight. Reaching your goal of a healthy lifestyle will help protect your heart for a lifetime.

We thank you for your continued support and dedication to women's heart health!

Ann M. Taubenheim, Ph.D., M.S.N.
Project Director, *The Heart Truth*
National Institutes of Health, National Heart, Lung, and Blood Institute

For instructions to make this heart-shaped sachet, see page 140. ➤

Crafting with care

Crafters know how fulfilling it is to use your hands to create something beautiful—and it's even more gratifying when your creation is part of a worthwhile cause. I've always found joy in crafting, and crochet has been a particular favorite: in home economics class in high school, when we were told to make a potholder, I crocheted an entire afghan! I love making things with my own hands, and then giving my handmade creations to people I care about. My daughter snuggles in her Mommy-made crochet afghan every night!

In addition to that feeling of creativity and accomplishment, repetitive activities like crochet have been shown to help lower your blood pressure and heart rate and reduce stress, important factors in maintaining heart health. That's particularly important to me, as I have a family history of heart disease.

In *Crochet Red* you'll find not only stunning designs, but a wealth of information and tips about heart health. Did you know that even though 80 percent of women said they would call 911 if they thought someone else was having a heart attack, barely half actually call 911 if they believe they're having a heart attack themselves? Statistics like that are alarming. The good news is that most heart disease is preventable, and women can reduce their risk by leading a heart-healthy lifestyle.

Use this book to raise awareness about heart disease among the women in your own life. Crochet some of these projects for your family and friends to remind them to take care of their own heart health.

The best thing we can do for the people we love is to make sure we stay healthy ourselves. With this book in hand, you can pick up your crochet hook knowing you're helping to improve the heart health of yourself and other women.
Could there be a better excuse to get crocheting?

❤ Deborah Norville

Give heart disease the hook

I learned to crochet when I was five years old, sitting with my grandmother Albertene Nicholas, and I still think of her every time I crochet a starting chain for a new project. I've crocheted gifts for every member of my family, and now my daughter, Giovanna, whom I taught to crochet when she was young, is carrying on the tradition.

For me, crochet is not just a hobby. It's about family togetherness and a connection to something greater than just the yarn. That's a big reason I was so excited for the opportunity to be a part of the community providing designs for this wonderful book.

Finding a cure for heart disease is such an important cause, and one that's been close to my heart my whole life. When I was a kid, my mom would work around the clock one weekend a year at a local radio station, WNMB in South Carolina, raising money to fight heart disease. I've always been involved in giving back to the community, and it's very special to be a part of the same cause for which my mother once fought so valiantly.

I am so grateful that heart disease does not run in my family. Still, I know I should never take my health for granted, and I take care of myself physically, mentally, and emotionally. A well-balanced diet and age-appropriate exercise are crucial for every woman, regardless of her genetics. In addition to what we put on our plates, keeping fit, getting enough sleep, and managing stress are critical to staying healthy and preventing disease. Plus, the meditative effect of yarn crafting is an exercise for the mind.

I'm devoted to maintaining an all-around healthy lifestyle not just for me, but for my children. Consider your loved ones as you educate yourself in healthy living and disease prevention, and understand the power one woman with a voice can have in saving the lives of friends and family. Start small. Pick up some red yarn and know that your choice to crochet red is increasing awareness of heart disease.
What are you waiting for?

❤ Vanna White

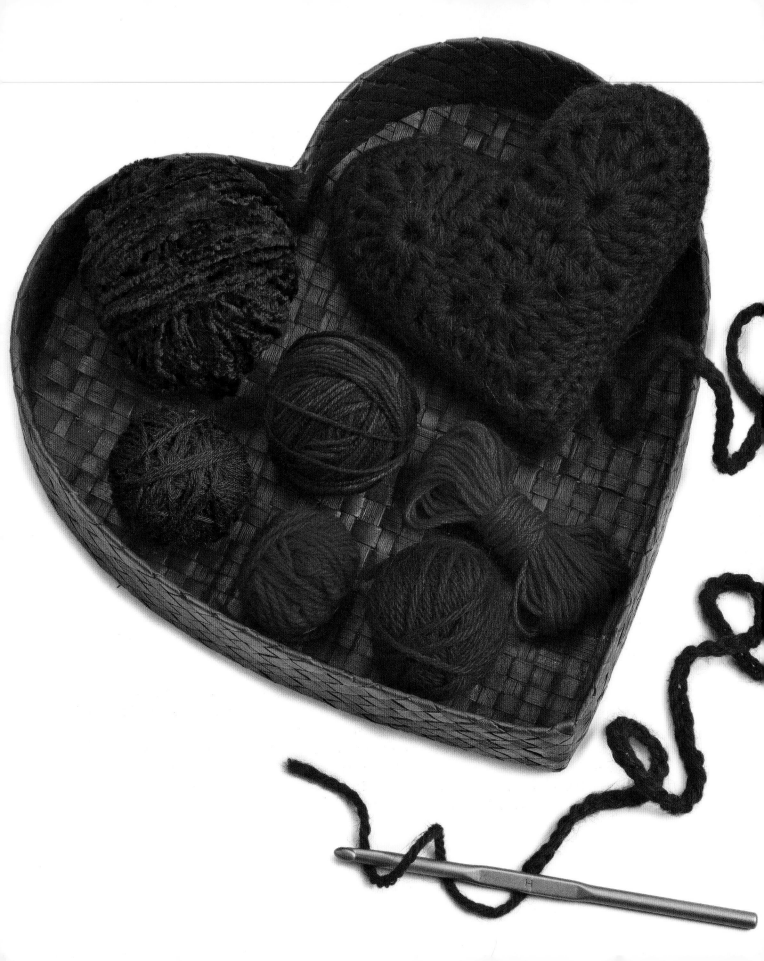

Stick it to heart disease!

If this book has made its way into your hands, it is because a) you love to crochet, b) you care about "sticking it to heart disease," or c) both! Whatever the reason, we thank you and hope you find it inspiring. Our goal with the Stitch Red campaign was to create awareness of heart disease, especially in women, through some of our favorite pastimes: crochet, knitting, and sewing. With the help of superstar designers, fabric and yarn producers, and our many friends in the crochet, knitting, sewing, and quilting worlds, the campaign has grown into an international crusade.

The Stitch Red campaign was born out of a shared experience with my friend Marta McGinnis in 2007. That year my husband, Doug, was diagnosed with high blood pressure, and Marta survived a major heart attack, which she subsequently found out was due to heart disease. Both Doug and Marta were otherwise healthy: they led active lifestyles and were, we thought, unusually young for the onset of heart problems (Marta was barely fifty; Doug was in his thirties). Marta and I dug deeper and were shocked to discover that heart disease is responsible for the deaths of more women than all cancers combined and kills more women than men each year. With the raw truth before us, we had to do something to raise awareness about this epidemic. Tragically, Marta passed away just six months later. Without her enthusiasm and encouragement, the Stitch Red campaign would not exist. Thank you, Marta—we miss you and hope we've made you proud.

After we released *Knit Red* in 2012, the overwhelming response from the crochet community was *What about crochet?* Not to worry, fellow crafters; we always planned on a crochet installment in the Stitch Red saga. After all, I was a crocheter before I was a knitter! Jimmy Beans Wool owes its existence in part to crochet: it was on a hunt for angora yarn to crochet a scarf for my mother that I stumbled into my first local yarn shop and became entranced and obsessed with yarn—an obsession that ended up taking over my daily life. To this day, crochet holds a special place in my heart. In fact, I nearly abandoned knitting when my son, Huck, was born in favor of crocheting beanie after beanie for him.

Crochet Red is a product of the crochet celebrities who donated their time, designs, and personal experiences with heart disease. We could not be more grateful. We also owe huge thanks to the dozens of companies who developed products specifically for the Stitch Red campaign and generously agreed to donate a portion of the proceeds from the sale of those products to the Foundation for the National Institutes of Health in support of *The Heart Truth*®. We hope that the designs and information in these pages will inspire you—to create, to share the word with others, and, most important, to care for your heart. ❤

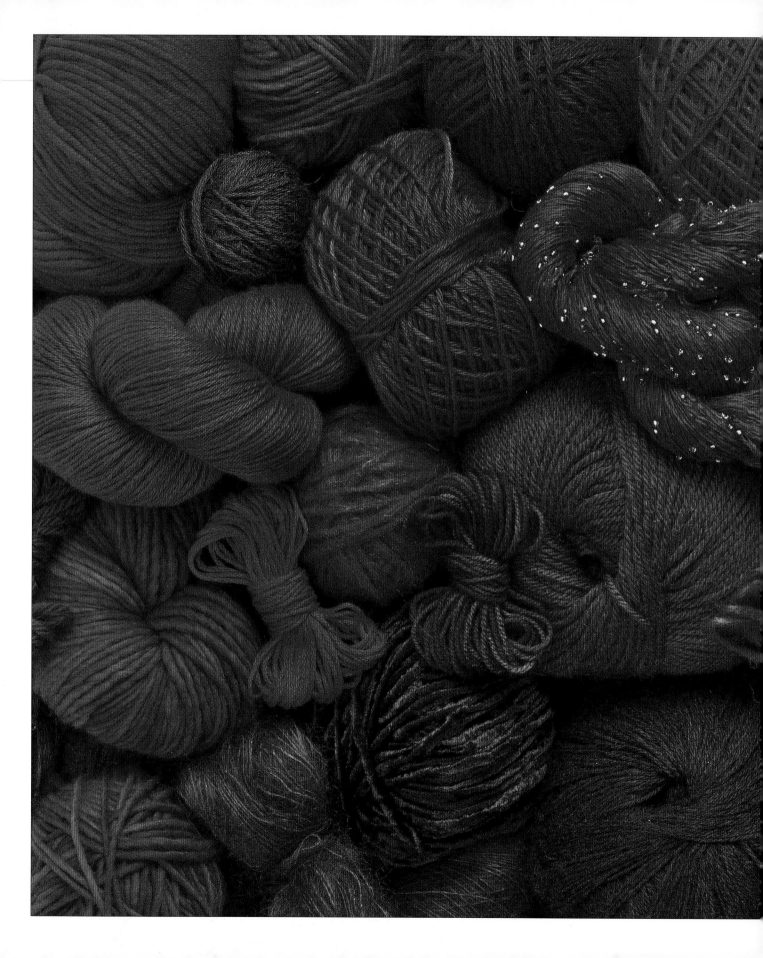

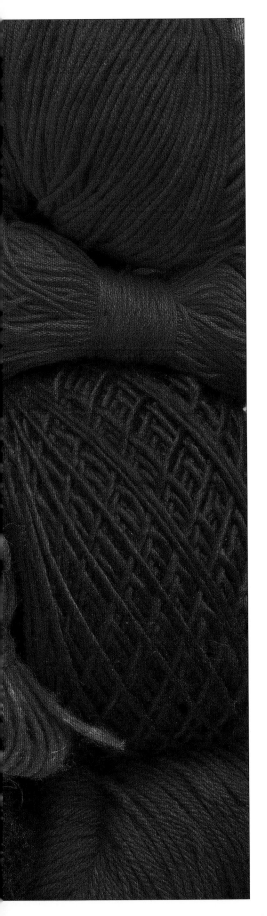

projects and profiles

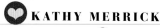

Peplum Jacket

A button-down jacket with a flattering peplum shape features a pretty border pattern repeated at the collar, waist, sleeves, buttonband, and bottom.

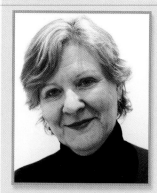

SIZES
Instructions are written for size X-Small. Changes for Small, Medium, Large, and X-Large are in parentheses. (Shown in size Small.)

MEASUREMENTS
BUST (BUTTONED)
28½ (33, 36½, 40¾, 44½)"/72.5 (84, 93.5, 103.5, 113)cm
LENGTH
23 (24, 25, 26, 27)"/58.5 (61, 63.5, 66, 68.5)cm

MATERIALS
• 4 (5, 6, 7, 8) 3½oz/100g hanks (each approx 525yd/480m) of Swans Island Company *Natural Colors Collection Fingering* (organic merino) in garnet
• Size D/3 (3.25mm) crochet hook *or size to obtain gauge*
• 6 (6, 7, 7, 8) buttons, ¾"/2cm diameter

GAUGE
28 sts and 14 rows = 4"/10cm over body pat using size D/3 (3.25mm) crochet hook.
➤ Take time to check gauge.

STITCH GLOSSARY
Cl (cluster) [Yo, pull up an extended lp in indicated st or sp] 4 times; yo and draw through all 9 lps on hook, ch 1.

BORDER PATTERN
(multiple of 12 sts plus 3, ch 1 extra for foundation)
Set-up row 1 Sc in 2nd ch from hook; *ch 1, sk next ch, sc in next ch; rep from * to end.
Set-up row 2 Sc in first sc, *ch 1, sk next ch-1 sp, sc in next sc; rep from * to end.
Row 1 Ch 1, sc in first sc, ch 1, sk next ch-1 sp, sc in next sc; *ch 5, sk next 2 ch-1 sps, sl st in next ch-1 sp 2 rows below, ch 5, sk 2 ch-1 sps, sc in next sc, ch 1, sc in next sc; rep from * to end.
Row 2 Ch 1, sc in first sc, ch 1, sk ch-1 sp, sc in next sc; *[ch 1, sk ch-1 sp, dc in next skipped sc of prev row] 4 times, ch 1, sc in next sc, ch 1, sk next ch-1 sp, sc in next sc; rep from * to end.
Rep rows 1 and 2 for border pat.

BODY PATTERN
(multiple of 4 sts plus 1, beg set-up with 2 extra sts)
Set-up row 1 Sc in 1st sc, (ch 3, cl) in same st, sk 4 sts, (sc, ch 3, cl) in next st, *sk 3 sts, (sc, ch 3, cl) in next st, rep from * to last 5 sts, sk 4 sts, sc in last st.
Set-up row 2 Ch 3, cl in first sc, (sc, ch 3, cl) in each ch-3 sp to last sp, sc in last sp.
Row 1 Ch 3, cl in first sc, (sc, ch 3, cl) in each sp to end.

Row 2 Ch 3, cl in first ch-3 sp, (sc, ch 3, cl) in each sp to last sp, sc in last sp.
Rep rows 1 and 2 for body pat.

NOTE
Jacket is worked in one piece back and forth to underarm, then divided for fronts and back.

BODY
HIP
Ch 220 (244, 268, 292, 316), and work set-up rows 1 and 2 of border pat.
Work rows 1 and 2 of border pat 4 (4, 5, 6, 6) times, then work row 1 once more.
Next row (WS) Ch 1, sc in each sc and ch-1 sp across—219 (243, 267, 291, 315) sts.
Work set-up rows 1 and 2 of body pat, then work rows 1 and 2 of body pat until piece measures 6½ (7, 7½, 8, 8½)"/16.5 (18, 19, 20.5, 21.5)cm, ending after a pat row 1.
Next row (WS) Ch 1, work 171 (195, 219, 243, 267) evenly across row.

WAIST
Work set-up row 2 of border pat twice.
Work rows 1 and 2 of border pat 5 (5, 6, 6, 7) times, then work row 1 once more.
Next row (WS) Ch 1, work 189 (221, 245, 273, 297) evenly across row.

KATHY'S STORY
Kathy Merrick wanted to be an artist when she grew up, a childhood aspiration that turned out quite accurate. With a great eye for color, Kathy creates stunning works of art using yarn as her canvas. Because of the way she collects different yarns and weaves them together in striking and often daring color combinations, Kathy jokingly calls herself a magpie—she's not afraid to play with seemingly mismatched shades and is attracted to bright colors that others might shy away from. Her adventurous style and deftness with color inspired a spectacular book, *Crochet in Color: Techniques and Designs for Playing with Color.* That's exactly what Kathy encourages crocheters to do: play! She loves to teach others to find inspiration and experiment with color in their crafting. Kathy's father suffered from rheumatic fever as a child, which later led to heart disease; his struggle inspired her to get on board with the Stitch Red campaign.

♥ KATHY'S TIP
TAKE ADVANTAGE OF YOUR SURROUNDINGS! Kathy takes long walks in the beautiful Morris Arboretum and Fairmount Park in nearby Philadelphia.

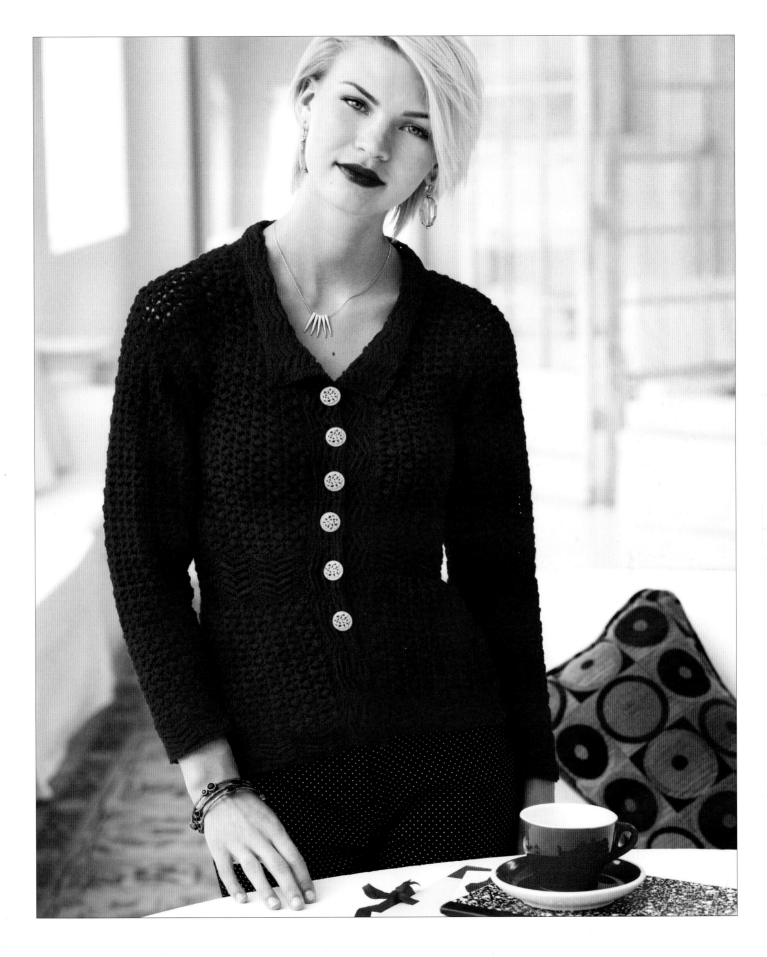

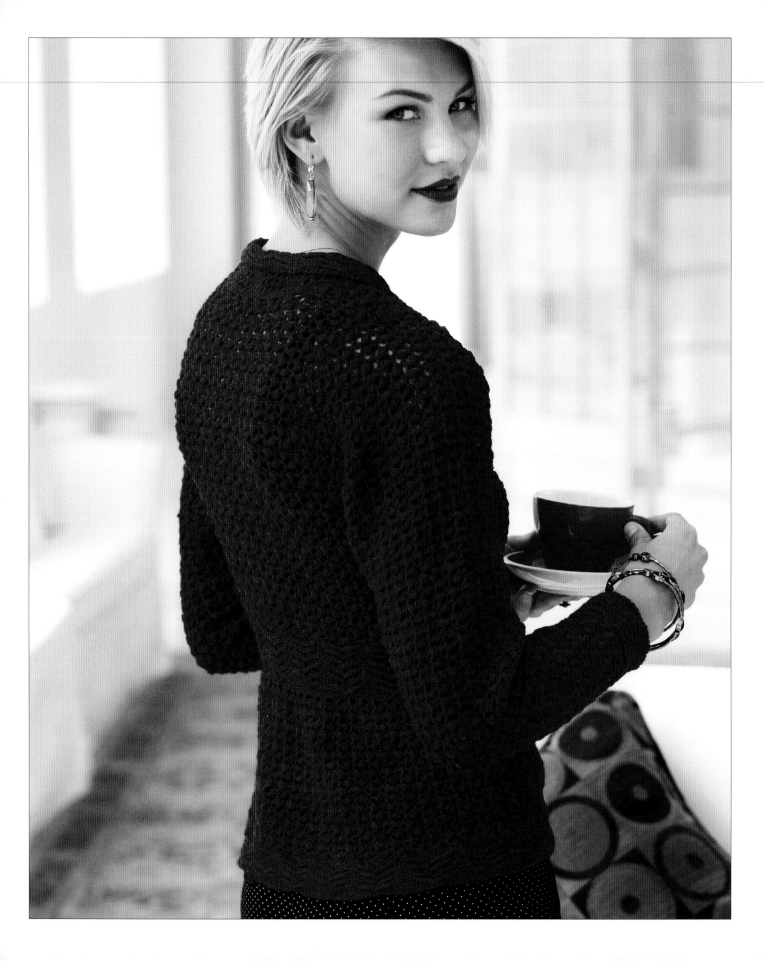

BUST

Work set-up rows 1 and 2 of body pat, then work rows 1 and 2 of body pat until piece measures 15 (15½, 16, 16½, 17)"/38 (39.5, 40.5, 42, 43)cm, ending after a pat row 2. Separate for back and fronts as foll:

RIGHT FRONT

Row 1 (RS) Ch 3, cl in first sc, *(sc, ch 3, cl) in next sp; rep from * 8 (10, 11, 13, 15) times more, turn.
Row 2 Work as body pat row 2—9 (11, 12, 14, 16) cl.
Row 3 Ch 3, cl in first sc, (sc, ch 3, cl) in each sp to last sp, sc in last sp—9 (11, 12, 14, 16) cl.
Row 4 Rep row 2—8 (10, 11, 13, 15) cl.
Row 5 Rep row 3—8 (10, 11, 13, 15) cl.
Row 6 Work as body pat row 2. Work even in body pat until armhole measures 4½ (4½, 5, 5, 5½)"/11.5 (11.5, 12.5, 12.5, 14)cm, ending after a body pat row 1.

NECK SHAPING

Row 1 (WS) Ch 3, cl in first ch-3 sp, *(sc, ch 3, cl) in next sp; rep from * 1 (2, 3, 4, 5) times more, turn.
Row 2 Ch 3, cl in first ch-3 sp, *(sc, ch 3, cl) in next sp; rep from * 1 (2, 3, 4, 5) times more.
Row 3 Work as body pat row 2. Work even in body pat until armhole measures 8 (8½, 9, 9½, 10)"/20.5 (21.5, 23, 24, 25.5)cm, ending after a body pat row 1. Fasten off.

BACK

With RS facing, sk 4 ch-3 sps at right underarm, and join yarn in next sc.
Row 1 (RS) Ch 3, cl in same sc as join, *(sc, ch 3, cl) in next sp; rep from * 17 (20, 25, 28, 30) times more, turn—19 (22, 27, 30, 32) cl.

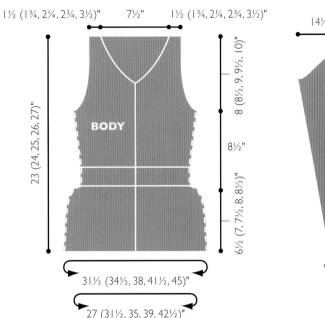

1½ (1¾, 2¼, 2¾, 3½)" 7½" 1½ (1¾, 2¼, 2¾, 3½)"

8 (8½, 9, 9½, 10)"

8½"

6½ (7, 7½, 8, 8½)"

23 (24, 25, 26, 27)"

BODY

31½ (34½, 38, 41½, 45)"

27 (31½, 35, 39, 42½)"

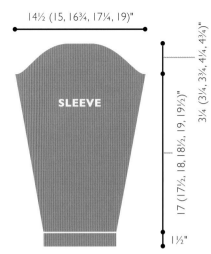

14½ (15, 16¾, 17¼, 19)"

SLEEVE

3¾ (3¾, 4, 4¼, 4¾)"

17 (17½, 18, 18½, 19, 19½)"

1½"

Row 2 Ch 3, cl in first ch-3 sp, (sc, ch 3, cl) in each sp to last sp, sc in last sp—18 (21, 26, 29, 31) cl.
Rows 3–5 Rep row 2—15 (18, 23, 26, 28) cl.
Row 6 Work as body pat row 2. Work even in body pat until armhole measures 8 (8½, 9, 9½, 10)"/20.5 (21.5, 23, 24, 25.5)cm, ending after a body pat row 1. Fasten off.

LEFT FRONT

With RS facing, sk 4 ch-3 sps at right underarm, and join yarn in next sc.
Row 1 (RS) Ch 3, cl in same sc as join, *(sc, ch 3, cl) in next sp; rep from * to end.
Row 2 Work as body pat row 2—9 (11, 12, 14, 16) cl.
Row 3 Ch 3, cl in first ch-3 sp, *(sc, ch 3, cl) in next sp; rep from * to end—9 (11, 12, 14, 16) cl.
Row 4 Rep row 2—8 (10, 11, 13, 15) cl.
Row 5 Rep row 3—8 (10, 11, 13, 15) cl.
Row 6 Work as body pat row 2. Work even in body pat until armhole measures 4½ (4½, 5, 5, 5½)"/11.5 (11.5, 12.5, 12.5, 14)cm, ending after a body pat row 2.

NECK SHAPING

Row 1 (RS) Ch 3, cl in first sc, *(sc, ch 3, cl) in next sp; rep from * 2 (3, 4, 5, 6) more times, turn.
Row 2 Work as body pat row 2.
Row 3 Ch 3, cl in first sc, *(sc, ch 3, cl) in next sp; rep from * 1 (2, 3, 4, 5) times more.
Row 4 Work as body pat row 2. Work even in body pat until armhole measures 8 (8½, 9, 9½, 10)"/20.5 (21.5, 23, 24, 25.5) cm, ending after a body pat row 1. Fasten off.

SLEEVE

Ch 52 (52, 64, 64, 64), and work set-up rows 1 and 2 of border pat.
Work rows 1 and 2 of border pat 4 (4, 5, 6, 6) times, then work row 1 once more.
Next row (WS) Ch 1, work 53 (57, 61, 65, 69) sc evenly across row.
Work set-up rows 1 and 2 of body pat and cont as foll:

Rows 1–4 Work in body pat.
Rows 5–7 Work as body pat row 1—15 (16, 17, 18, 19) cl.
Row 8 Work as body pat row 2. Rep rows 1–8 for 5 (5, 6, 6, 7) times more, then work a body pat row 1—25 (26, 29, 30, 33) cl. Work even in body pat until sleeve measures 18½ (19, 19½, 20, 20½)"/47 (48.5, 49.5, 51, 52)cm, ending after a body pat row 1.

CAP SHAPING

With WS facing, sk 2 ch-3 sps, and join yarn in next sc.
Row 1 (WS) Ch 3, cl in next ch-3 sp, *(sc, ch 3, cl) in next sp; rep from * to last 2 sps, sk last 2 sps, turn.
Work 1 (1, 1, 3, 3) more rows evenly in body pat—21 (22, 25, 26, 29) cl.
Next 9 (9, 11, 11, 13) rows (beg and end WS) Work as body pat row 2—12 (13, 14, 15, 16) cl. Fasten off.

FINISHING

Sew back to fronts at shoulders.

BUTTON BAND

With RS facing, work 87 (93, 99, 105, 111) sc down left front edge.

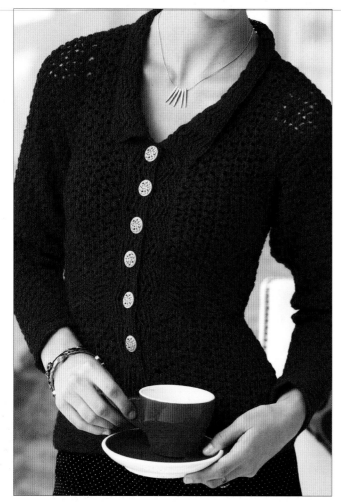

Sizes X-Small, Medium, and X-Large only

Next row (WS) Ch 1, sc in first sc, *ch 1, sk 1 sc, sc in next sc; rep from * to end.

Work rows 1 and 2 of border pat 4 (5, 6) times, then work row 1 once more.

Next row Ch 1, sc in each sc and ch-1 sp across. Fasten off.

Sizes Small and Large only

Next 3 rows:

Row 1 (WS) Ch 1, sc in each of the first 2 sc, *ch 1, sk 1 sc, sc in next sc; rep from * to last sc, sc in last sc.

Row 2 Ch 1, sc in each of the first 2 sc, ch 1, sk next ch-1 sp, work row 1 of border pat to last 3 sts, ch 1, sk next ch-1 sp, sc in each of the last 2 sc.

Row 3 Ch 1, sc in each of the first 2 sc, ch 1, sk next ch-1 sp, work row 2 of border pat to last 3 sts, ch 1, sk next ch-1 sp, sc in each of the last 2 sc.

Rep the last 2 rows 3 (4) more times, then work row 2 only (as above) once more.

Next row Ch 1, sc in each sc and ch-1 sp across. Fasten off.

BUTTONHOLE BAND

With RS facing, work 87 (93, 99, 105, 111) sc up left front edge.

Sizes X-Small, Medium, and X-Large only

Next row (WS) Ch 1, sc in first sc, *ch 1, sk 1 sc, sc in next sc; rep from * to end.

Work rows 1 and 2 of border pat 2 (2, 3) times, then work row 1 once more.

Next row (WS) Ch 1, sc in first sc, *ch 3, sk ch-1 sp, sc in next sc, [ch 1, sk ch-1 sp, dc in next skipped sc of prev row] 4 times, ch 1, sc in next sc; rep from * 5 (6, 7) times, work in established pat to end.

Work rows 1 and 2 of border pat 1 (2, 3) times more, then work row 1 once more.

Next row Ch 1, sc in each sc and ch-1 sp across. Fasten off.

Sizes Small and Large only

Next 3 rows:

Row 1 (WS) Ch 1, sc in each of the first 2 sc, *ch 1, sk 1 sc, sc in next sc; rep from * to last sc, sc in last sc.

Row 2 Ch 1, sc in each of the first 2 sc, ch 1, sk next ch-1 sp, work row 1 of border pat to last 3 sts, ch 1, sk next ch-1 sp, sc in each of the last 2 sc.

Row 3 Ch 1, sc in each of the first 2 sc, ch 1, sk next ch-1 sp, work row 2 of border pat to last 3 sts, ch 1, sk next ch-1 sp, sc in each of the last 2 sc.

Rep last 2 rows 1 (2) times more, then work row 2 once more.

Next row (WS) Ch 1, sc in each of the first 2 sc, ch 1, sk next ch-1 sp, sc in next sc, *ch 3, sk ch-1 sp, sc in next sc, [ch 1, sk ch-1 sp, dc in next skipped sc of prev row] 4 times, ch 1, sc in next sc; rep from * 5 (6, 7) times, work in established pat to end.

Work rows 2 and 3 as above 1 (2, 3) times more, then work row 2 once more.

Next row Ch 1, sc in each sc and ch-1 sp across. Fasten off.

COLLAR

With RS facing, work 159 (171, 183, 195, 207) sc evenly around neck edge.

Work set-up row 2 of border pat.

Work rows 1 and 2 of border pat 8 (8, 9, 9, 10) times, then work row 1 once more.

Next row (WS) Ch 1, sc in each sc and ch-1 sp across. Fasten off.

Using mattress stitch, sew sleeves in armhole openings of body, easing in extra fabric as needed. Sew sleeve seams. Sew buttons opposite buttonholes. Block lightly to measurements. ❤

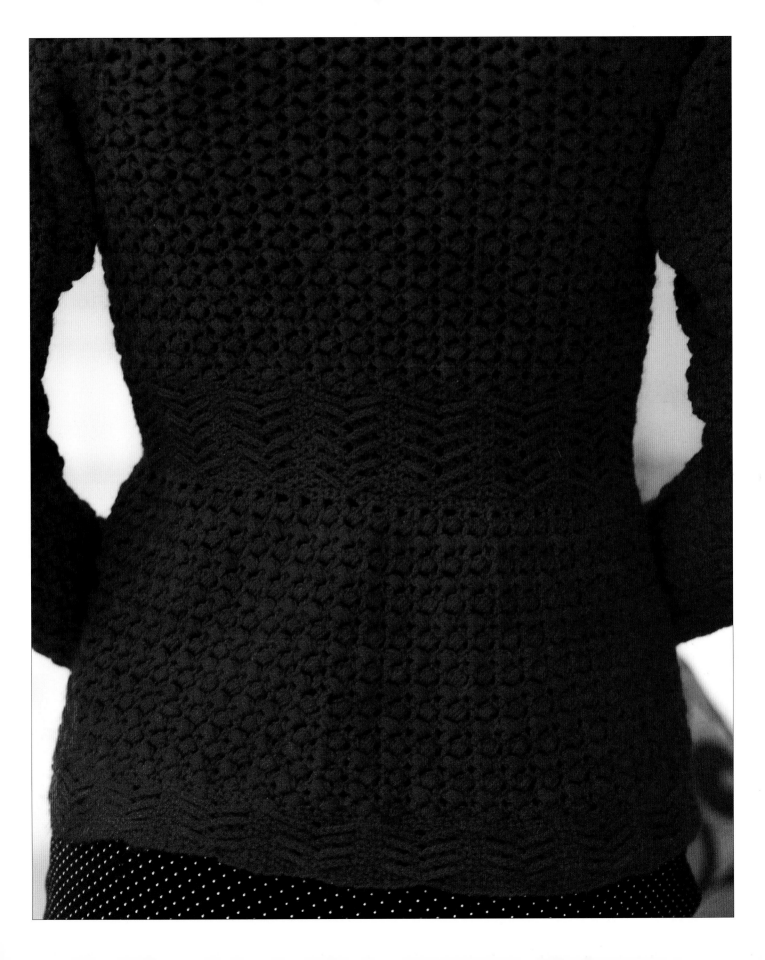

Bobble & Check Cowl

The stitch pattern changes from checks to bobbles halfway through this generously sized cowl, adding textural interest to an easy-to-crochet piece.

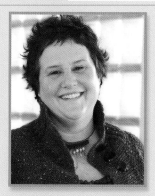

■■□□

SIZE
Instructions are written for one size.

MEASUREMENTS
CIRCUMFERENCE
66"/167.5cm
WIDTH
8"/20.5cm

MATERIALS
• 3 3½oz/100g hanks (each approx 217yd/198m) of Berroco Vintage (acrylic/wool/nylon) in #5150 berries (4)
• Size G/6 (4mm) crochet hook or size to obtain gauge
• Tapestry needle

GAUGE
20 sts and 10 rows = 4"/10cm over buttonhole check pat using size G/6 (4mm) crochet hook.
➤ Take time to check gauge.

STITCH GLOSSARY
bob (4-hdc bobble) Ch 4, *yo, insert hook around post of prev sc just made and draw up a lp; rep from * 3 times more around *same* sc, yo and draw through all 9 lps on hook, ch 1.

rev sc (reverse single crochet) Insert hook into indicated sp or st in opposite direction as you normally crochet (right-hand crocheters insert hook in next st to the right; left-hand crocheters insert hook in next st to the left). Draw up a lp, yo and draw through 2 lps on hook.

COWL
Ch 44.

BUTTONHOLE CHECK PATTERN SECTION
Row 1 (RS) Dc in 4th ch from hook (sk ch counts as dc), *dc in next 4 ch, sk 1 ch, ch 1; rep from * to last 5 ch, dc in last 5 ch—34 dc.
Row 2 Ch 1, turn, sc in first dc, *ch 4, sk 4 dc, sc in ch-1 sp; rep from * to last 5 sts, ch 4, sc in top of t-ch.
Row 3 Ch 3 (counts as dc), turn, *4 dc in ch-4 sp, ch 1, sk sc; rep from * to last ch-4 sp, 4 dc in last ch-4 sp, dc in last sc.
Rep rows 2 and 3 until piece measures 32"/81.5cm long, ending with a row 2.

♥ NORAH'S TIP
TRY TO GET IN A DAILY WALK FOR EXERCISE, and take the stairs instead of the elevator whenever possible. Especially on the way up!

Next row Ch 3, turn, 5 dc in first ch-4 sp, 4 dc in each ch-4 sp across, dc in last sc—35 dc.

BOBBLE ARCH PATTERN SECTION
Row 1 Ch 1, turn, sc in first dc, *sc in next dc, bob around prev sc, sk 2 dc; rep from * to t-ch, sc in top of t-ch—11 bob.
Row 2 Ch 3 (counts as dc), turn, 3 dc in each ch-4 sp (on top of bob) across, dc in last sc—35 dc.
Rep rows 1 and 2 until piece measures 66"/167.5cm long, ending with a row 2.

FINISHING
Block lightly to measurements.

JOIN ENDS
Fold cowl in half, placing RS together, matching foundation ch with last row. Join yarn to end with sl st, working through both layers at once. Ch 1, sc in same st, *ch 4, sk 4 sts, sc in next st; rep from * across, ch 4, sc in last st, fasten off.

Join yarn to one edge of cowl, working around row ends on edge, rev sc evenly around, sl st to first rev sc, fasten off. Rep on opposite edge. ♥

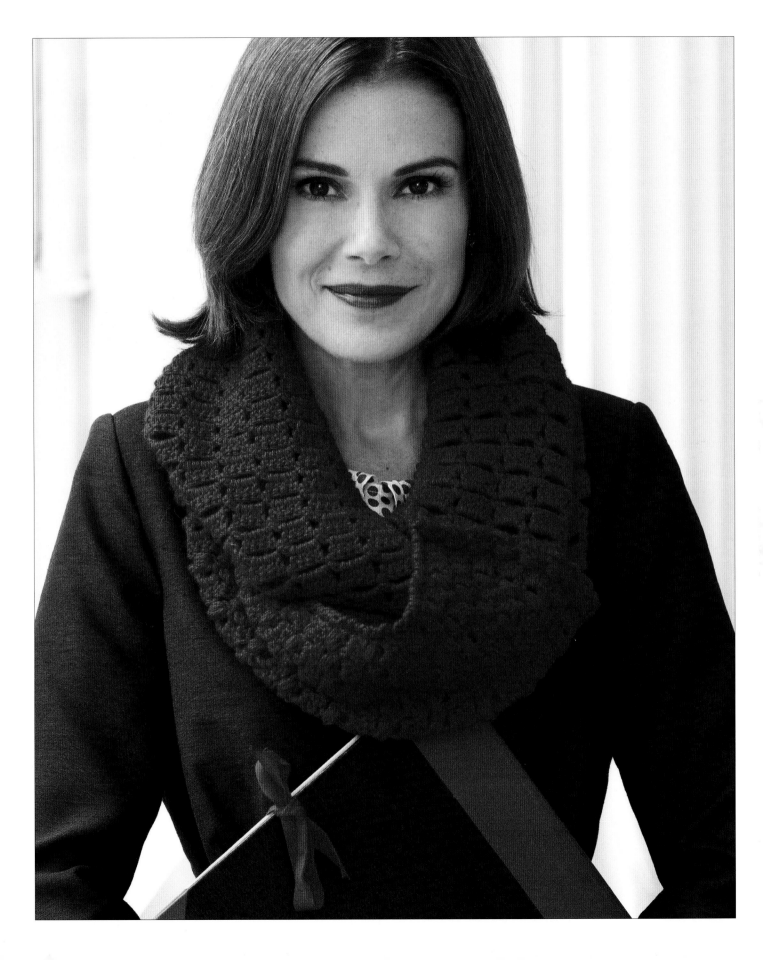

Woven Cardigan

The geometry of this cropped cardigan is defined by a tonal stripe pattern that goes horizontal on the back panel.

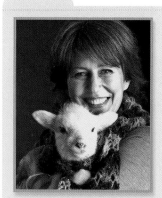

SIZES
Instructions are written for size Small. Changes for Medium and Large are in parentheses. (Shown in size Medium.)

MEASUREMENTS
BACK WIDTH
20 (22½, 25½)"/51 (57, 65)cm
LENGTH
15 (16, 18)"/38 (40.5, 45.5)cm

MATERIALS
• 2 (3, 3) 3½oz/100g hanks (each approx 252yd/230m) of Hamilton Yarns *Heaven's Hand Silke* (silk) in crimson (A) **(4)**
• 2 (3, 3) 3½oz/100g skeins (each approx 219yd/200m) of Hamilton Yarns *Heaven's Hand Wool Classic* (wool) in red (B) **(4)**
• Size I/9 (5.5mm) crochet hook *or size to obtain gauge*

GAUGE
18 sts and 16 rows = 4"/10cm over stripe pat using size I/9 (5.5mm) crochet hook.
➤Take time to check gauge.

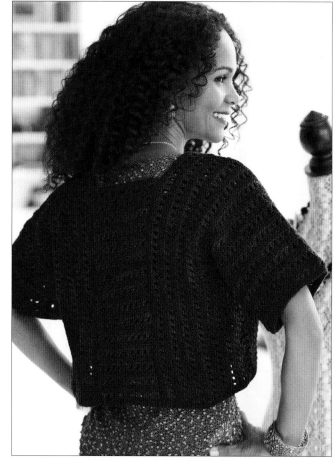

STRIPE PATTERN
(over an odd number of sts)
Rows 1 and 2 (beg RS) Using A, ch 1, sc in each st to end.
Row 3 Using B, ch 3 (counts as 1 dc), *ch 1, sk next sc, dc in next sc, rep from * to end.
Row 4 Using B, ch 1, sc in first dc, *sc in next ch-1 sp, sc in next dc; rep from * to end.
Rep rows 1–4 for stripe pat.

RIGHT SLEEVE AND BODY
Using A, ch 68 (72, 84).
Row 1 (RS, counts as first row of stripe pat) Sc in 2nd ch from hook and in each ch to end—67 (71, 83) sc.
Work 19 more rows in stripe pat, beg with pat row 2—5 pat reps completed.

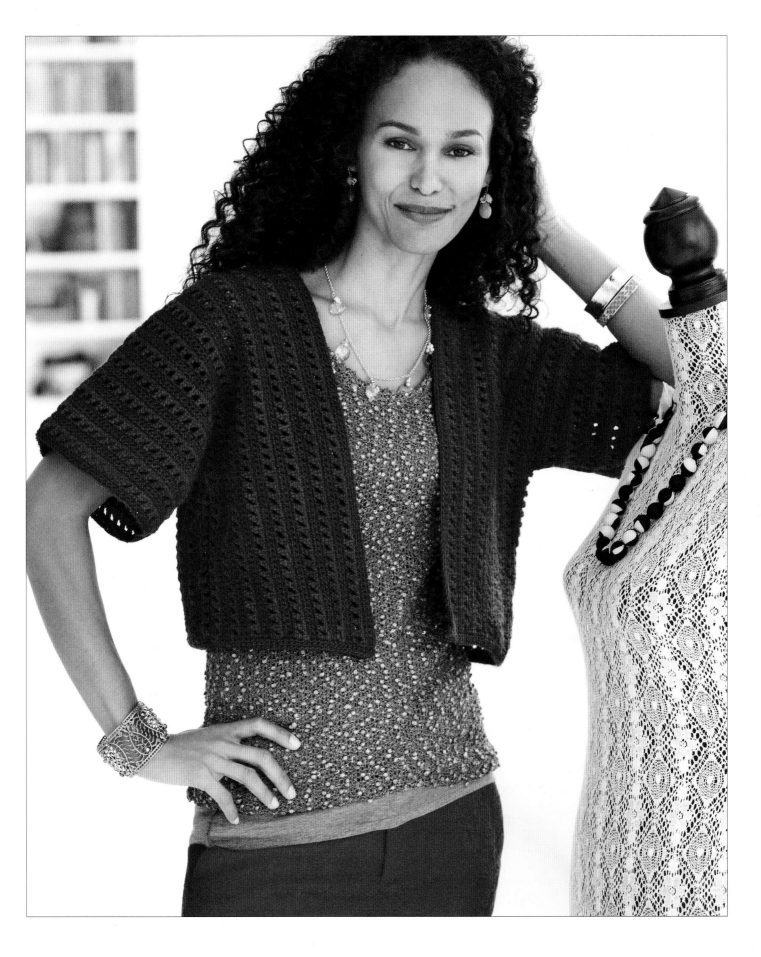

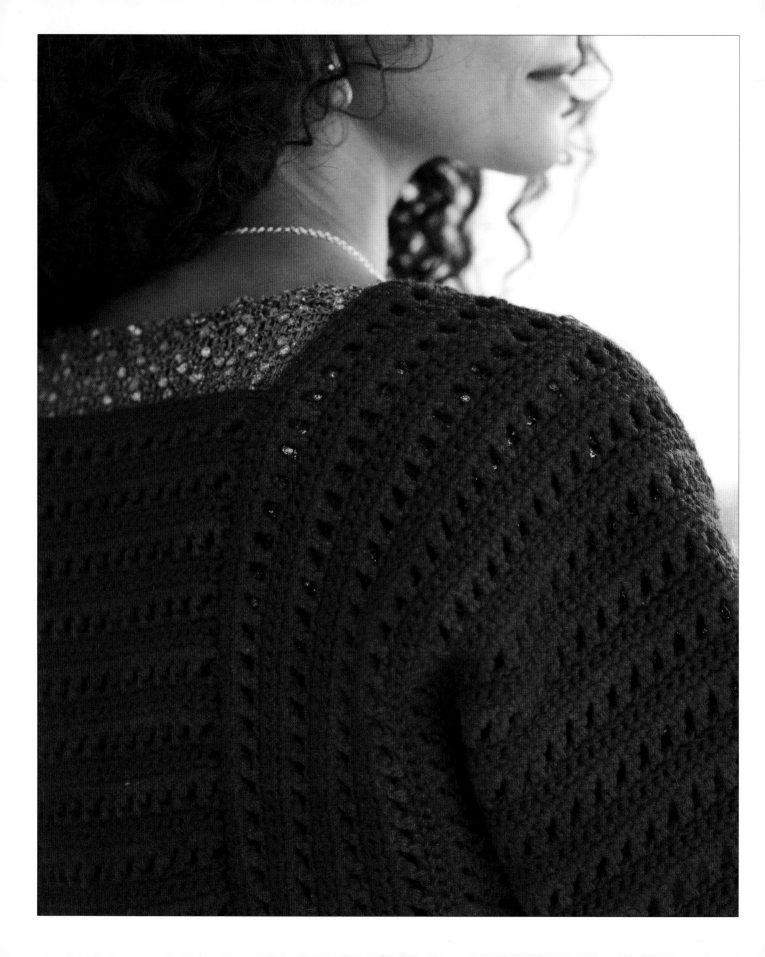

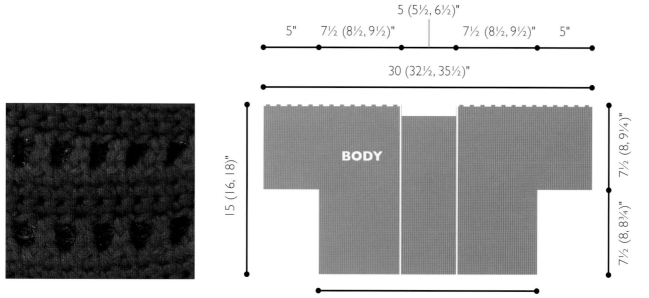

5 (5½, 6½)"

5"   7½ (8½, 9½)"   7½ (8½, 9½)"   5"

30 (32½, 35½)"

BODY

15 (16, 18)"

7½ (8, 9¼)"

7½ (8, 8¾)"

20 (22½, 25½)"

Row 21 (RS) Ch 35 (37, 41), sc in 2nd ch from hook and in each ch to sleeve sts, sc in next dc, *sc in next ch-1 sp, sc in next dc; rep from * to end.
Row 22 Ch 35 (37, 41), sc in 2nd ch from hook and in each ch to sleeve sts, sc in each sc to end—135, 143, 163 sts. Work 28 (32, 36) more rows in stripe pat as established—12½ (13½, 14½) pat reps completed from beg. Fasten off.

LEFT SLEEVE AND BODY
Work as for right sleeve and body.

BACK PANEL
Using A, ch 24 (26, 30).
Row 1 (RS, counts as first row of stripe pat) Sc in 2nd ch from hook and in each ch to end—23 (25, 29) sc.

Work 57 (61, 69) more rows in stripe pat, beg with pat row 2—14½ (15½, 17½) pat reps completed. Fasten off.

FINISHING
Join side and sleeve seams. Place back panel between the right and left body pieces. Pin or baste pieces together, starting at lower edge and making sure the stripes stay horizontal. Join back panel to body pieces.

BOTTOM EDGING
Work 2 rows in sc evenly across entire bottom edge.❤

♥**CORNELIA'S TIP**
DON'T BE A FANATIC ABOUT COUNTING CALORIES, but choose the best fuel for your body: coconut oil over animal fats; more veggies and organic foods and less wheat and dairy.

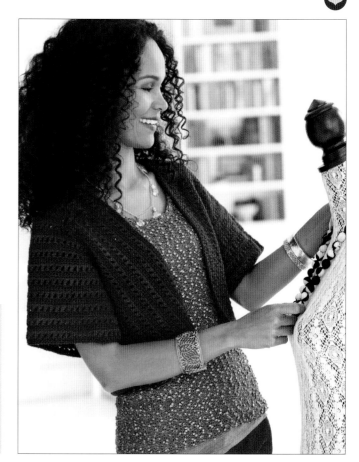

SHARON H. SILVERMAN

Tunisian Chevron Scarf

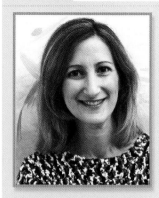

Worked in Tunisian crochet, this scarf uses a simple chevron pattern to let the dimensionality of the luscious chenille yarn take center stage.

MEASUREMENTS
WIDTH 5"/12.5cm
LENGTH 63"/160cm

MATERIALS
• 5 1¾oz/50g balls (each approx 61yd/56m) of Muench Yarns *Touch Me* (rayon/wool) in #3620 maroon (4)
• Size K/10½ (6.5mm) Tunisian crochet hook *or size needed to obtain gauge*

GAUGE
25 sts and 13 rows = 5"/12.5cm over Tunisian simple st using size K/10½ (6.5mm) Tunisian crochet hook.
➤ Take time to check gauge.

STITCH GLOSSARY
M1 (make 1) Inc by pulling up a lp in horizontal strand before next vertical bar and pull it snug to hook. Gently stretch sts apart to find this strand.
RP (return pass) Ch 1, *yo and draw through 2 lps; rep from * until 1 lp rem on hook.
Tss (Tunisian simple stitch) Pull up a lp in next vertical bar.

NOTES
1) This is a Tunisian crochet pattern. Each row is worked in two passes: the forward pass, which adds loops onto the hook, and the return pass, which works loops off the hook. The right side is always facing you. Never turn your work.
2) The first loop on hook counts as first stitch of each row. Do not work into the first vertical bar.
3) For the final stitch on each forward pass, insert the hook behind two strands of yarn, the vertical bar and the horizontal thread that runs behind it— looked at from the side, it will resemble a backward "6."
4) To join yarns, start a new ball of yarn on the final stitch of a return pass. Simply drop the old yarn and work the last stitch from the new ball.
5) Practice a few rows of the pattern on smooth, light-colored yarn before using the chenille.

SCARF
Ch 25.
Row 1 (RS) Pull up a lp in 2nd ch from hook and in each ch to end—25 lps on hook. RP.
Row 2 M1, tss in each of next 7 sts, yo and draw through 3 lps, tss in each of next 4 sts, M1, tss in next st, M1, tss in each of next 7 sts, yo and draw through 3 lps, tss in each of next 4 sts, M1, tss in last st—25 lps on hook. RP.
Rep row 2 until scarf measures approx 62½"/159cm.
Next row Sc in each vertical bar across.
Fasten off.

FINISHING
Block lightly to measurements. ❤

SHARON'S STORY
She's a successful designer and author with six books under her belt, but Sharon Silverman didn't set out to be a crochet guru. As a child, she wanted to be a veterinarian, and when her mother tried to teach her to knit, it didn't go well. Neither did her attempts at embroidery; she once cross-stitched a pillowcase to her pants! But when she picked up a crochet hook, it was a match made in heaven. She was working as a freelance travel writer when an editor asked her to contribute to a new line of craft books, and before she knew it, she had embarked on a design career. We're glad she did! Sharon knows that education is important in preventing heart disease; she joined the Stitch Red campaign to help keep crafters informed about healthy lifestyles. Like many of us, she has several friends and family members who have been affected by the disease, including one who underwent a heart transplant. Sharon takes care of her heart by playing tennis—she'd play every day if she could—and keeping fresh veggies on steady rotation in her diet.

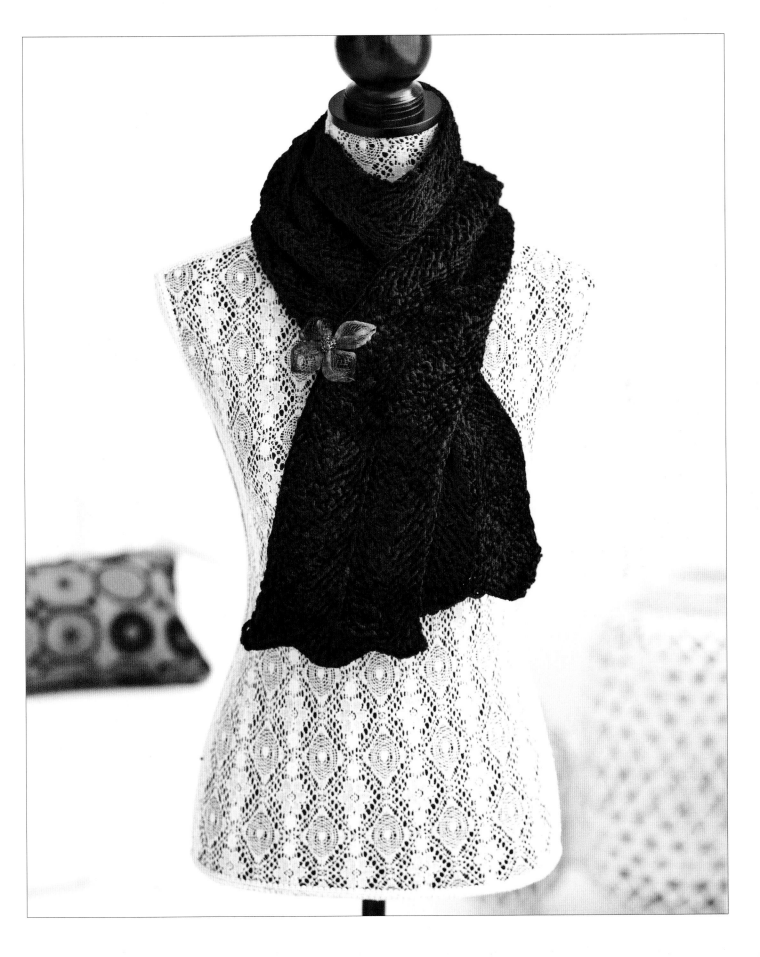

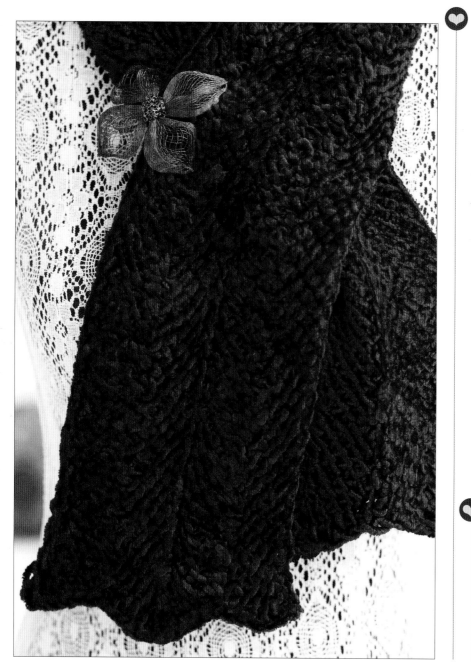

♥**SHARON'S TIP**
A FAVORITE MEAL
OF SHARON'S is
delicious and heart-healthy
bruschetta: a whole-grain
baguette toasted and
rubbed with garlic, then
piled with fresh tomatoes
and basil and drizzled with
olive oil—yum!

STITCH KEY

◯ ch

+ sc

⊓̃ Tss

⌣ MI

↻ Yo and draw
through 3 lps

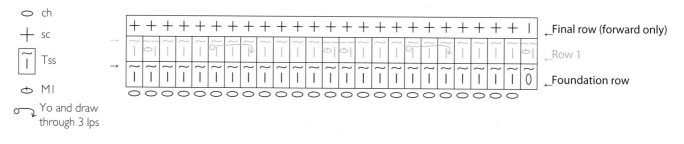

←Final row (forward only)

Row 1

←Foundation row

♥ LINDA PERMANN

Petal Cabled Hat

Pretty petals transform into cables that flow toward the brim of this soft, slightly oversized alpaca hat, which works up quickly from the top down.

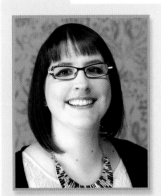

LINDA'S STORY
A full-time Craftsy instructor and the author of three books and hundreds of designs, Linda Permann breaks the mold of the granny square—but she'll teach you to crochet one! She picked up a hook in her early twenties and taught herself the craft, and now combines her training as an artist with a passion for teaching—she loves designing classes as much as garments. Linda also experiments with other crafts like knitting, sewing, and making jewelry. She keeps things light (calling her father a member of the "zipper club," due to his heart surgery scar), but knows that her family history requires her to focus on diet and exercise. Luckily, she loves to walk, and takes her Chihuahua, Freddie, on two outings daily—it's convenient and easy to fit a few minutes of walking into even a hectic day.

SIZE
Instructions are written for one size.

MEASUREMENTS
BRIM CIRCUMFERENCE
22"/56cm
HEIGHT 8"/20.5cm

MATERIALS
• 2 1¾oz/50g skeins (each approx 120yd/109m) of Blue Sky Alpacas *Techno* (alpaca/silk/merino) in #1976 cha-cha red (5)
• Size G/7 (4.5mm) crochet hook *or size to obtain gauge*
• Tapestry needle

GAUGE
4 rnds = 3¾"/9.5cm over st pat, unblocked, using size G/7 (4.5mm) crochet hook.
➤ Take time to check gauge.

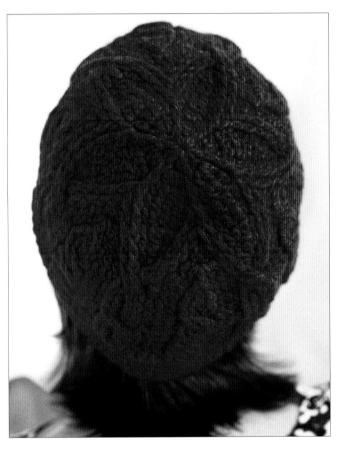

STITCH GLOSSARY
dc2tog (double crochet 2 together) [Yo, insert hook in next st and pull up a lp, yo and draw through 2 lps on hook] twice, yo and draw through all 3 lps on hook.

dc3tog (double crochet 3 together) [Yo, insert hook in next st and pull up a lp, yo and draw through 2 lps on hook] 3 times, yo and draw through all 4 lps on hook.

FPdc (front-post double crochet) Yo, insert hook from front to back and then to front again around post of indicated st, yo and pull up lp, [yo and draw through 2 lps on hook] twice.

FPtr (front-post treble crochet) [Yo] twice, insert hook from front to back and then to front again around post of indicated st, yo and pull up lp, [yo and draw through 2 lps on hook] 3 times.

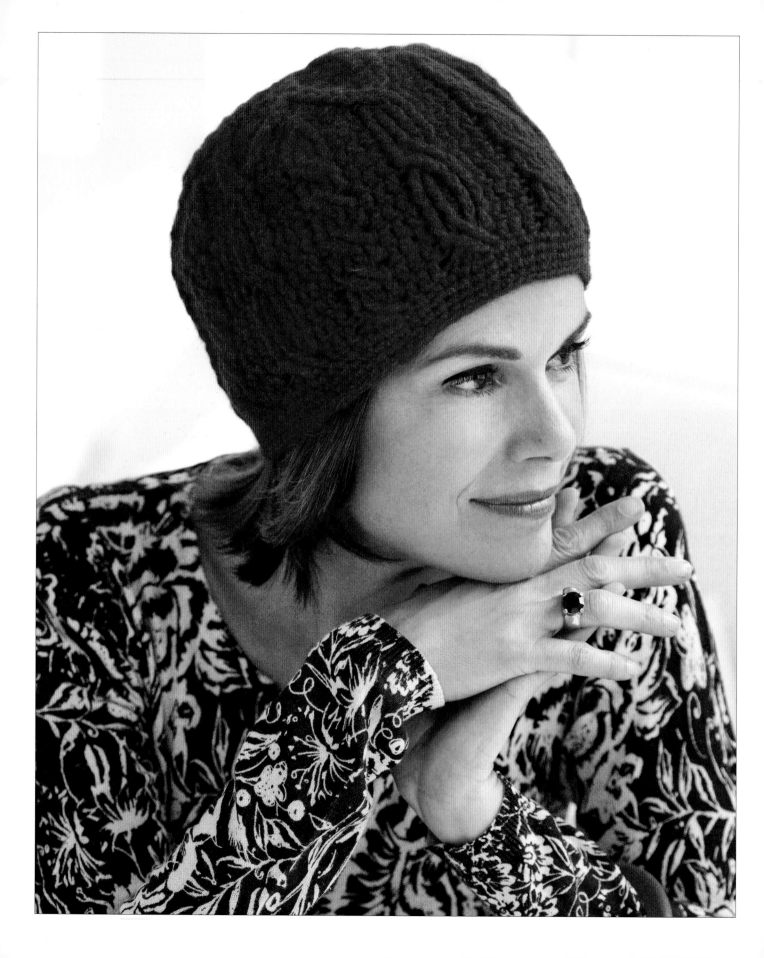

Cable cross Sk next 3 sts, FPtr around each of next 2 FPdc; working behind the FPtr sts just made, dc in skipped dc; working in front of the FPtr stitches just made, FPtr around first skipped FPdc, FPtr around next skipped FPdc.

sc2tog (single crochet 2 together) [Insert hook in next st and draw up a lp] twice, yo and draw through all 3 lps on hook.

NOTE

When instructed to work (FPdc, dc, FPdc) around a st, work the first FPdc around the st, the dc into the top of the st, and the last FPdc around the st.

HAT

Make an adjustable ring.

Rnd 1 (RS) Ch 3 (counts as first dc here and throughout), 11 dc in ring; join with sl st in top of beg-ch—12 dc.

Rnd 2 Ch 2 (does not count as a st here and throughout), FPdc around first dc (the beg ch-3), 3 dc in next dc, [FPdc around next dc, 3 dc in next dc] 5 times; join with sl st in top of beg-ch—18 dc and 6 FPdc.

Rnd 3 Ch 2, [FPdc around next FPdc, dc in next dc, 2 dc in next dc, dc in next dc] 6 times; join with sl st in top of beg-ch—24 dc and 6 FPdc.

Rnd 4 Ch 2, [(FPdc, dc, FPdc) around next FPdc, dc in next 4 dc] 6 times; join with sl st in top of beg-ch—30 dc and 12 FPdc.

Rnd 5 Ch 2, [FPdc around next FPdc, (FPdc, dc, FPdc) around next dc, FPdc around next FPdc, dc in next 4 dc] 6 times; join with sl st in top of beg-ch—30 dc and 24 FPdc.

Rnd 6 Ch 2, [FPdc around each of next 2 FPdc, 3 dc in next dc, FPdc around each of next 2 FPdc, dc in next dc, dc2tog, dc in next dc] 6 times; join with sl st in top of beg-ch—36 dc and 24 FPdc.

Rnd 7 Ch 2, [FPdc around each of next 2 FPdc, dc in next dc, 3 dc in next dc, dc in next dc, FPdc around each of next 2 FPdc, dc in next 3 dc] 6 times; join with sl st in top of beg-ch—48 dc and 24 FPdc.

Rnd 8 Ch 2, [FPdc around each of next 2 FPdc, 2 dc in next dc, dc in next dc, (FPdc, dc, FPdc) around next dc, dc in next dc, 2 dc in next dc, FPdc around each of next 2 FPdc, dc3tog] 6 times; join with sl st in top of beg-ch—48 dc and 36 FPdc.

Rnd 9 Sl st in each of next 2 FPdc, sl st in next dc, ch 3 (counts as first dc here and throughout), dc in next 2 dc, FPdc around next FPdc, (FPdc, dc, FPdc) around next dc, FPdc around next FPdc, dc in next 3 dc, cable cross, [dc in next 3 dc, FPdc around next FPdc, (FPdc, dc, FPdc) around next dc, FPdc around next FPdc, dc in next 3 dc, cable cross] 5 times; join with sl st in top of beg-ch—42 dc, 24 FPdc and 6 cable crosses.

Rnd 10 Ch 3, dc in next 2 dc, FPdc around each of next 2 FPdc, dc in next dc, FPdc around each of next 2 FPdc, dc in next 3 dc, FPdc around each of next 2 FPtr; dc in next dc, FPdc around each of next 2 FPtr, [dc in next 3 dc, FPdc around each of next 2 FPdc, dc in next dc, FPdc around each of next 2 FPdc, dc in next 3 dc, FPdc around each of next 2 FPtr; dc in next dc, FPdc around each of next 2 FPtr] 5 times; join with sl st in top of beg-ch—48 dc and 48 FPdc.

Rnd 11 Ch 3, dc in next 2 dc, cable cross, dc in next 3 dc, FPdc around each of next 2 FPdc, dc in next dc, FPdc around each of next 2 FPdc, [dc in next 3 dc, cable cross, dc in next 3 dc, FPdc around each of next 2 FPdc, dc in next dc, FPdc around each of next 2 FPdc] 5 times; join with sl st in top of beg-ch—42 dc, 24 FPdc, and 6 cable crosses.

Rnd 12 Ch 3, dc in next 2 dc, FPdc around each of next 2 FPtr; dc in next dc, FPdc around each of next 2 FPtr; dc in next 3 dc, FPdc around each of next 2 FPdc, dc in next dc, FPdc around each of next 2 FPdc, [dc in next 3 dc, FPdc around each of next 2 FPtr; dc in next dc, FPdc around each of next 2 FPtr; dc in next 3 dc, FPdc around each of next 2 FPdc, dc in next dc, FPdc around each of next 2 FPdc] 5 times; join with sl st in top of beg-ch—48 dc and 48 FPdc.

Rnd 13 Rep rnd 11.

Rnd 14 Ch 3, dc in next 2 dc, FPdc around each of next 2 FPtr; dc in next dc, FPdc around each of next 2 FPtr; dc in next 3 dc, cable cross, [dc in next 3 dc, FPdc around each of next 2 FPtr, dc in next dc, FPdc around each of next 2 FPtr; dc in next 3 dc, cable cross] 5 times; join with sl st in top of beg-ch—42 dc, 24 FPdc and 6 cable crosses.

Rnd 15 Ch 3, dc in next 2 dc, cable cross, dc in next 3 dc, FPdc around each of next 2 FPtr; dc in next dc, FPdc around each of next 2 FPtr; [dc in next 3 dc, cable cross, dc in next 3 dc, FPdc around each of next 2 FPtr; dc in next dc, FPdc around each of next 2 FPtr] 5 times; join with sl st in top of beg-ch—42 dc, 24 FPdc, and 6 cable crosses.

Rnds 16 and 17 Rep rnds 12 and 13.

Rnd 18 Rep rnd 12.

Rnd 19 Ch 3, dc in next 2 dc, cable cross, [dc in next 3 dc, cable cross] 11 times; join with sl st in top of beg-ch—36 dc and 12 cable crosses.

Rnd 20 Ch 1, sc in same st as joining, sc2tog, [sc in next 6 sts, sc2tog] 11 times, sc in last 5 sts; join with sl st in first sc—84 sc.

Rnds 21–23 Ch 1, sc in each sc around; join with sl st in first sc. Fasten off.

FINISHING

Block lightly to measurements. ❤

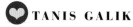

Gingham Afghan

A simple woven technique results in an oversized gingham pattern and fringed edges—a bit of Scottish elegance for the home.

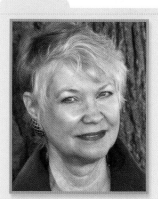

MEASUREMENTS
WIDTH 44"/111.5cm
LENGTH (NOT INCLUDING FRINGE) 50"/125cm

MATERIALS
• 8 3½oz/100g hanks (each approx 225yd/206m) of Madelinetosh *Tosh Merino DK* (superwash merino) in tart (A)
• 6 hanks in charcoal (B)
• Size J/10 (6mm) crochet hook *or size to obtain gauge*
• Tapestry needle

GAUGE
9 mesh boxes = 4"/10cm using size J/10 (6mm) crochet hook.
➤Take time to check gauge.

STRIPE PATTERN
Work [12 rows A, 12 rows B] 4 times, then 12 rows A.

AFGHAN
With A, ch 220.
Row 1 (RS) Dc in 6th ch from hook, [ch 1, skip next ch, dc in next ch] across, turn—108 ch-1 sps.
Row 2 Ch 4 (counts as dc, ch-1), [dc in next dc, ch 1] across. Dc in 4th ch of t-ch, turn.
Row 3 Ch 4, [dc in next dc, ch 1] across. Dc in 3rd ch of t-ch, turn.
Rows 4–108 Rep row 3 to desired length, changing color for stripe pat.

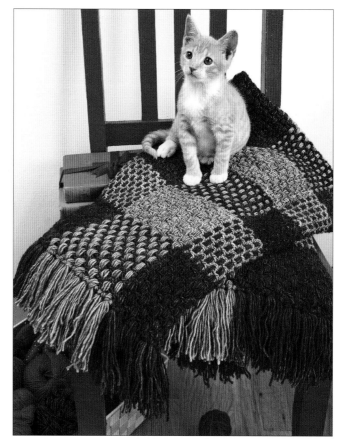

Fasten off when complete. Block lightly to measurements.

WEAVE PLAID
Rotate work 90 degrees. Cut 6 strands of A, each approx 62"/157.5cm long. Leaving a 6"/15cm tail on each end for fringe, weave yarn through the mesh, over the 1st dc and under the next. Rep for next row, working under the 1st dc and over the next. Follow same stripe pattern to create plaid design.

FINISHING
FRINGE
For each tail cut 6 strands of yarn, each approx 12"/30cm long, matching colors. Fold 6 strands in half, put loop through first mesh box, and thread all fringe and ends through loop. Gently pull fringe ends to tighten. Trim fringe to even lengths.♥

TANIS'S STORY
When we saw Tanis Galik's afghan design for *Crochet Red*, our response was: "You can do *that* with crochet?" Innovative and show-stopping designs are the trademark of this Northern California artist, who teaches for the Crochet Guild of America and is the author of the groundbreaking book *Interlocking Crochet*. Taught the basics of crochet by her grandmother at a young age, Tanis loves to use simple stitches to create a myriad of textures and looks in her designs. Tanis was shocked to learn that heart disease is the number-one killer of women, and immediately wanted to get involved in the Stitch Red campaign. We're elated that she agreed to use crochet to help spread the word! In her own life, Tanis prevents heart disease through exercise and healthy eating. She prefers to take her exercise outdoors: you can usually find her walking her two dogs or gardening.

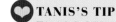 **TANIS'S TIP**
TANIS DOESN'T PROFESS TO BE AN EXCELLENT CHEF, but she does try to incorporate as many vegetables as possible into her cooking, like the fresh veggies in her favorite ham and vegetable soup.

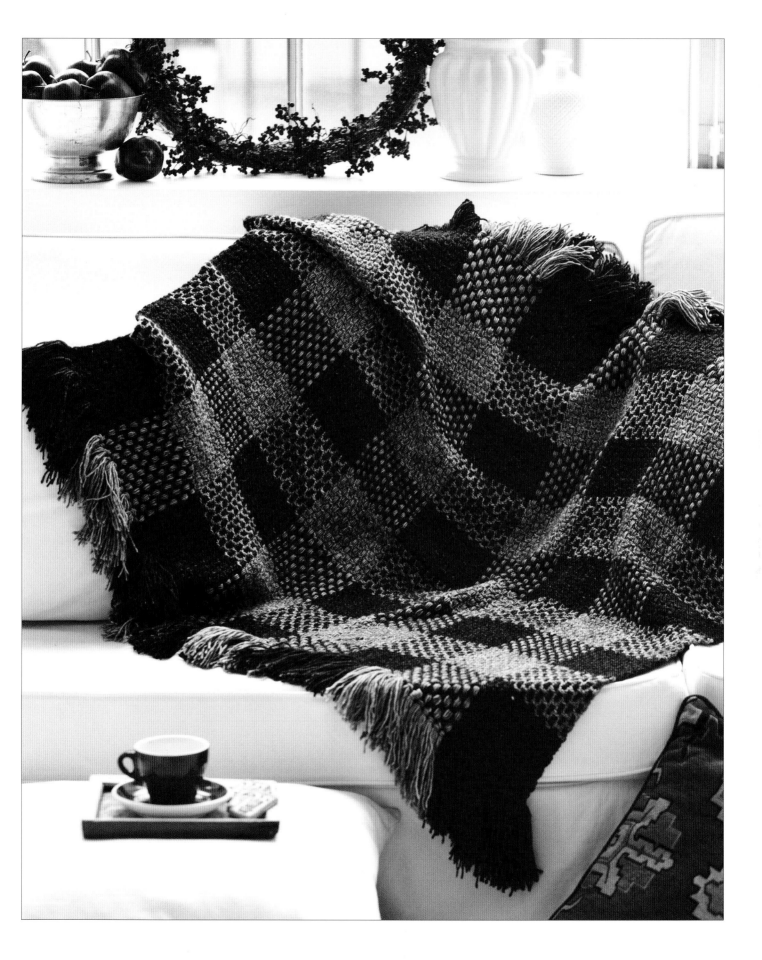

Tilting Blocks Shrug

A geometric block motif and sawtooth edging give a modern vibe to a romantic, feminine shrug that can be dressed up or down.

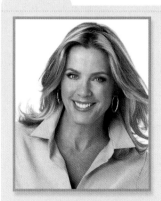

▬◀■■▭

SIZES
Instructions are shown for size Small/Medium. Changes for size Large/X-Large are in parentheses. (Shown in size Small/Medium.)

MEASUREMENTS
BUST 36 (44)"/91.5 (112)cm
ARM CIRCUMFERENCE 12 (14)"/30.5 (35.5)cm
LENGTH CUFF TO CUFF 54 (58)"/137 (147)cm

MATERIALS
• 3 (5) 4oz/113g skeins (each approx 203yd/186m) of Premier Yarns Deborah Norville Collection *Everyday Soft Worsted* (acrylic) in #1007 really red (4)
• Size H/8 (5mm) crochet hook *or size to obtain gauge*
• Tapestry needle

GAUGE
2 motifs and 4 rows = 4"/10cm square over tilting blocks pat using size H/8 crochet hook.
➤Take time to match gauge.

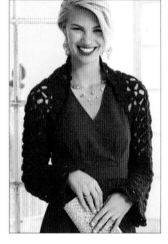

NOTES
1) Shrug is worked out from the center back to each cuff.
2) Sleeve length can easily be adjusted by working fewer or additional repeats of the tilting blocks pattern.

TILTING BLOCKS PATTERN
(multiple of 10 sts plus 1)
Row 1 Ch 4, [5 tr in ch-4 sp, sk 4 tr, tr in next tr, ch 4] to end of row, tr in top of t-ch, turn.
Rep row 1 for tilting blocks pat.

SHRUG
FIRST HALF
Ch 65 (75).
Row 1 Tr in 5th ch from hook and next 4 ch, sk 4 ch, tr in next ch, ch 4, [tr in next 5 ch, sk 4 ch, tr in next ch, ch 4] 5 (6) times, tr in next ch, turn—37 (43) tr and 6 (7) ch-sps.

Work in tilting blocks pat until piece measures 27 (29)"/68.5 (73.5)cm, fasten off.

SECOND HALF
Attach yarn in 1st st of foundation ch, work in base of ch.
Row 1 Ch 4, [5 tr in ch-4 sp, sk 4 ch, tr in next ch, ch 4] to last ch, tr in next ch.
Work in tilting blocks pat until piece measures 27 (29)"/68.5 (73.5)cm from foundation ch, fasten off.

FINISHING
Fold shrug in half lengthwise. Seam 12"/30.5cm at each end to form the sleeves, leaving the center 30 (34)"/76 (86.5)cm open.

EDGING
Join yarn at the center back.
Rnd 1 Sc evenly around center opening, working 3 sc in end of each row, sl st in 1st sc to join.
Rnd 2 [(Sc, ch 3, 3 dc) in next st, sk 2 sts] to end of rnd, sl st in 1st sc to join. Fasten off.

CUFF EDGING
Join yarn at seam.
Rnd 1 [4 sc in ch-4 sp, sc in next 5 tr] to end of rnd, sl st in 1st sc to join.
Rnd 2 [(Sc, ch 3, 3 dc) in next st, sk 2 sts] to end of rnd, sl st in 1st sc to join. Fasten off.
Repeat for second cuff.♥

DEBORAH'S STORY
You probably recognize Deborah Norville from the TV show *Inside Edition*, but you may not know she's also a popular knit and crochet designer, with her own line of yarns under the Premier brand. As a girl, Deborah knitted and crocheted doll clothes and afghans. She's a huge proponent of crafting as stress relief, which dramatically reduces blood pressure—a fun way to take care of your health! That's important to Deborah, due to her family history of heart problems: her father has high cholesterol and underwent a quintuple bypass, and her grandfather passed away from an aneurysm at sixty-eight. Deborah limits her sodium and cholesterol and cooks with fresh veggies, steaming or sautéing them to retain the vitamins. She also makes sure her family keeps red meat to a minimum and finds healthier substitutes for junk food, like crispy kale chips with garlic—who needs potato chips?

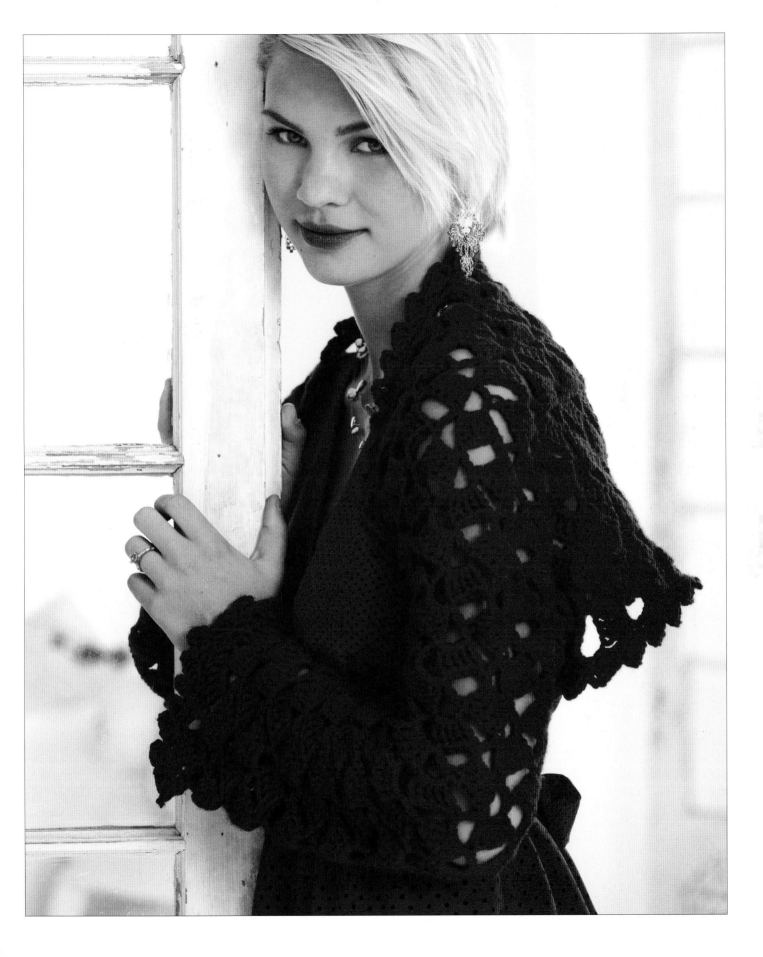

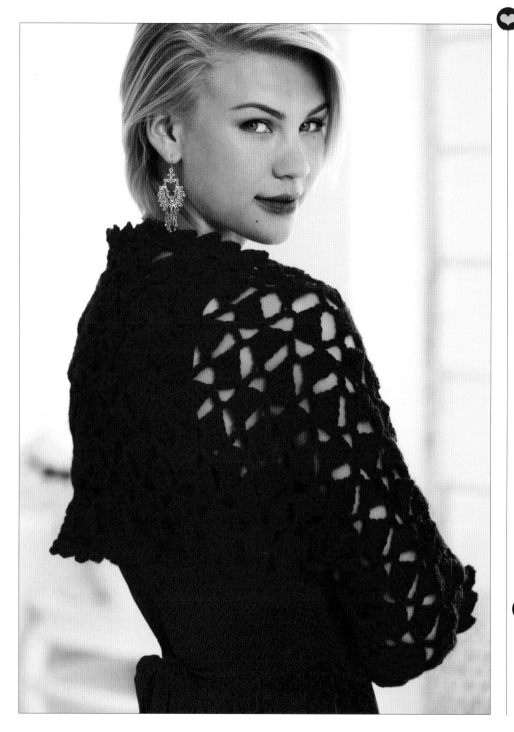

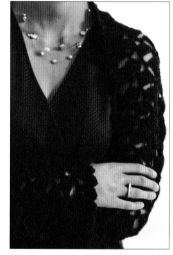

♥ **DEBORAH'S TIP**
KEEP HEALTHY
SNACKS that are loaded
with protein, like raw
almonds, on hand at all
times. Make it easy to make
good choices!

54 (56)"

12 (14)"

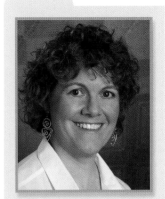

❤ EDIE ECKMAN

Slouchy Cowl

This beautifully draped cowl is a showcase of design details: a combination of puff clusters and V-stitches finished with a puff-stitch edging.

◼◼◻▭

SIZE
Instructions are written for one size.

MEASUREMENTS
CIRCUMFERENCE
33"/84cm
HEIGHT
7"/18cm

MATERIALS
• 1 3½oz/100g hank (each approx 241yd/220m) of Fyberspates *Scrumptious DK Worsted* (silk/merino) in #100 cherry red (❹)
• Size I/9 (5.5mm) crochet hook *or size to obtain gauge*
• Tapestry needle

GAUGE
4 pat rep = 4½"/11.5cm and 8 rows = 4"/10cm using size I/9 (5.5mm) crochet hook.
➤ Take time to check gauge.

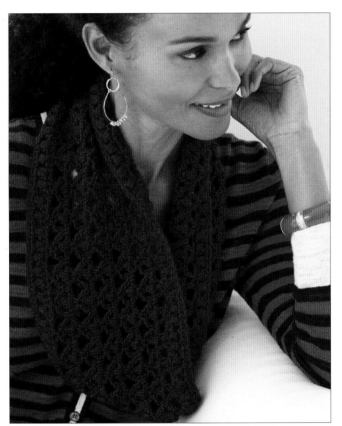

STITCH GLOSSARY
puff-Cl (puff cluster) Yo, insert hook in indicated sp and draw up a lp (3 lps on hook), [yo, insert hook in *same* sp and draw up a lp] twice (7 lps on hook), yo and draw through 6 lps on hook, yo and draw through 2 lps on hook.
puff-st Yo, insert hook in indicated st and draw up a lp (3 lps on hook), [yo, insert hook in same st and draw up a lp] twice (7 lps on hook), yo and draw through all 7 lps on hook.
V-st (Dc, ch 1, dc) in indicated st.

COWL
Ch 120 very loosely. Being careful not to twist ch, join with sl st in first ch to form a ring.
Rnd 1 (RS) Ch 4 (counts as dc, ch 1), dc in same st as joining (first V-st completed), *sk next 3 ch, V-st in next ch; rep from * around to last 3 ch, sk last 3 ch; join with sl st in 3rd ch of beg ch-4—30 V-sts.

EDIE'S STORY
Former yarn shop owner Edie Eckman turned to designing so she could focus on what she loves best: crochet! She learned at age six from her grandmother, who also taught Edie to knit, embroider, and sew. A career in fiber arts followed, and for over twenty years she's been designing, teaching, and editing crochet and knit patterns and techniques. Edie has written or collaborated on almost thirty books and teaches workshops on crochet, knitting, and pattern writing and editing. She's also a technical editor and a whiz at making charts! Edie had a good reason to be part of *Crochet Red* and the Stitch Red campaign: her grandfather died of a heart attack, and her father struggled with congestive heart failure. Edie is committed to living a healthy lifestyle to prevent problems with her own heart, so she practices yoga religiously and walks her dog every day.

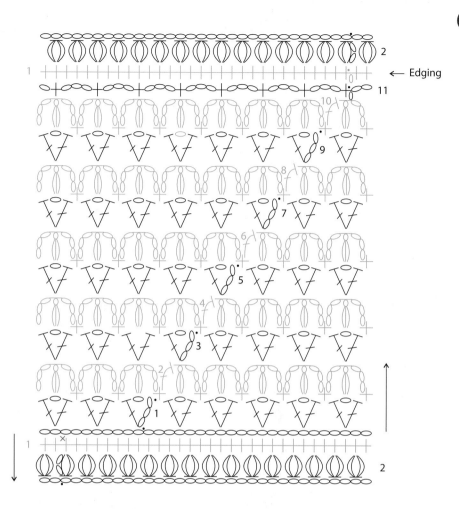

STITCH KEY

- •   sl st
- ◯   ch
- ┬   dc
- ⋎   V-st
- puff st
- puff cl
- ✕   Join with sl st
- ↑   Direction of work

Rnd 2 Ch 3, puff-Cl in first ch-1 sp, *ch 3, sc in next sp between V-sts, ch 3, puff-Cl in ch-1 sp of next V-st; rep from * around; join with dc in sp between last V-st and first V-st—30 puff-Cl.

Rnd 3 Ch 4, dc in top of joining dc, V-st in each puff-Cl around; join with sl st in 3rd ch of beg ch-4.

Rnd 4 Rep rnd 2.

Rnds 5–10 Rep rnds 3 and 4 three times more.

Rnd 11 Ch 1, sc in first puff-Cl, *ch 3, sc in next puff-Cl; rep from * around, ch 3; join with sl st in first sc. Do not fasten off.

EDGING

Rnd 1 Ch 1, sc in first sc, 3 sc in next ch-3 sp, *sc in next sc, 3 sc in next ch-3 sp; rep from * around; join with sl st in first sc—120 sc.

Rnd 2 Ch 2, puff-st in same st as joining, *ch 1, sk next 2 sc, puff-st in next sc; rep from * around to last 2 sc, ch 1, sk last 2 sc; join with sl st in top of first puff-st—40 puff-sts.
Fasten off.
Working across opposite side of foundation ch, draw up a lp in ch at base of any V-st, rep edging around.

FINISHING
Weave in ends. ❤

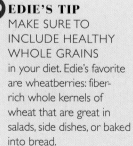

EDIE'S TIP
MAKE SURE TO INCLUDE HEALTHY WHOLE GRAINS in your diet. Edie's favorite are wheatberries: fiber-rich whole kernels of wheat that are great in salads, side dishes, or baked into bread.

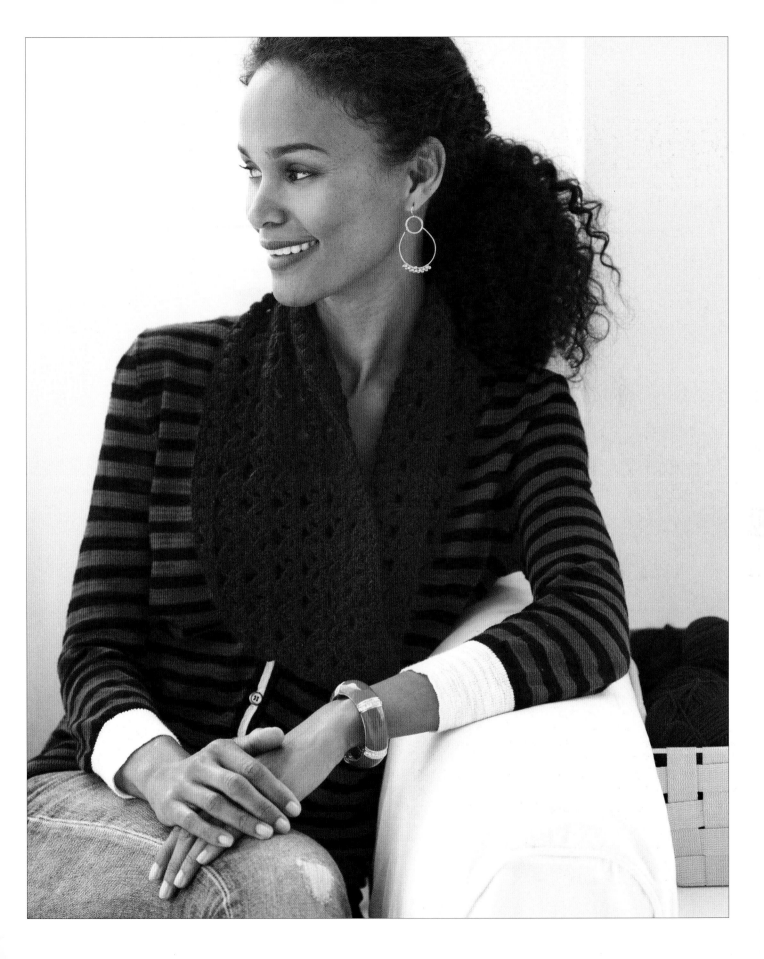

♥ ROHN STRONG

Vintage Tunisian Shell

A simple to memorize stitch pattern gives this airy summer shell its attractive drape. Make it in just a few hours to dress up or dress down.

SIZES
Instructions are written for size X-Small. Changes for Small, Medium, Large, and X-Large are in parentheses. (Shown in size Small.)

MEASUREMENTS
BUST
34 (36, 38, 42, 46)"/81 (86, 96.5, 101.5, 106.5)cm
LENGTH
16½ (17, 17, 18, 18)"/42 (43, 43, 45.5, 45.5)cm

MATERIALS
• 2 (2, 3, 3, 4) 3½oz/100g skeins (each approx 380yd/347m) of SweetGeorgia Yarns *Merino Silk Fine* (merino/silk) in cherry
• One each sizes H/8 and K/10½ (5 and 6.5mm) 14" Tunisian crochet hook *or size to obtain gauge*
• Tapestry needle

GAUGE
16 sts and 10 rows to 4"/10cm square over Tunisian double knit st with size K/10½ (6.5mm) Tunisian crochet hook after blocking.
➤ Take time to check gauge.

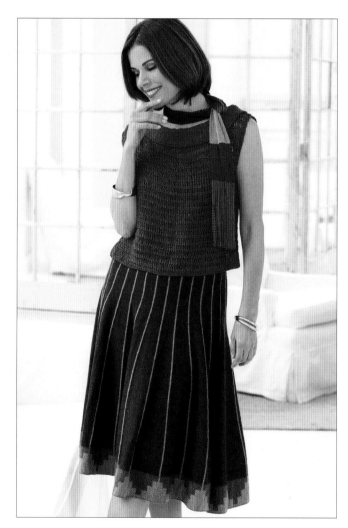

STITCH GLOSSARY
Tdks (Tunisian double knit stitch) Yo, insert hook through center of vertical bar (hook should pass under chain formed on return of previous row), yo, draw up a lp, yo and draw through 2 lps.

Tks (Tunisian knit stitch) Insert hook through center of vertical bar (hook should pass under chain formed by return of the previous row), yo and draw up a lp.

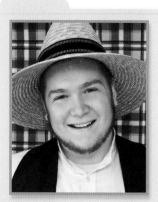

ROHN'S STORY
A crocheter since age six, North Carolina's Rohn Strong is an up-and-coming crochet and knitwear designer. His designs reflect not only a desire to push the boundaries of the craft, but also a personal connection to creating handmade items. Rohn uses crochet to combine his two favorite things: fiber arts and history! Rohn took his fascination with the two World Wars and created a book of patterns that any woman of those eras would have been proud to knit for her soldier, *The Heritage Collection: WWI & WWII*. He also headed up the Scarves for Soldiers project, collecting scarves knit from vintage patterns for the National WWII Museum in New Orleans. After being displayed, the scarves were donated to WWII veterans. Rohn didn't think twice about joining the Stitch Red campaign. Having watched his mother struggle with heart issues from a young age, he sees it as his duty to spread the word about the dangers of heart disease—and what better way than by doing what he loves best? He wants people to know that heart disease is usually preventable, and they can protect themselves by getting regular checkups, not smoking, and eating healthy.

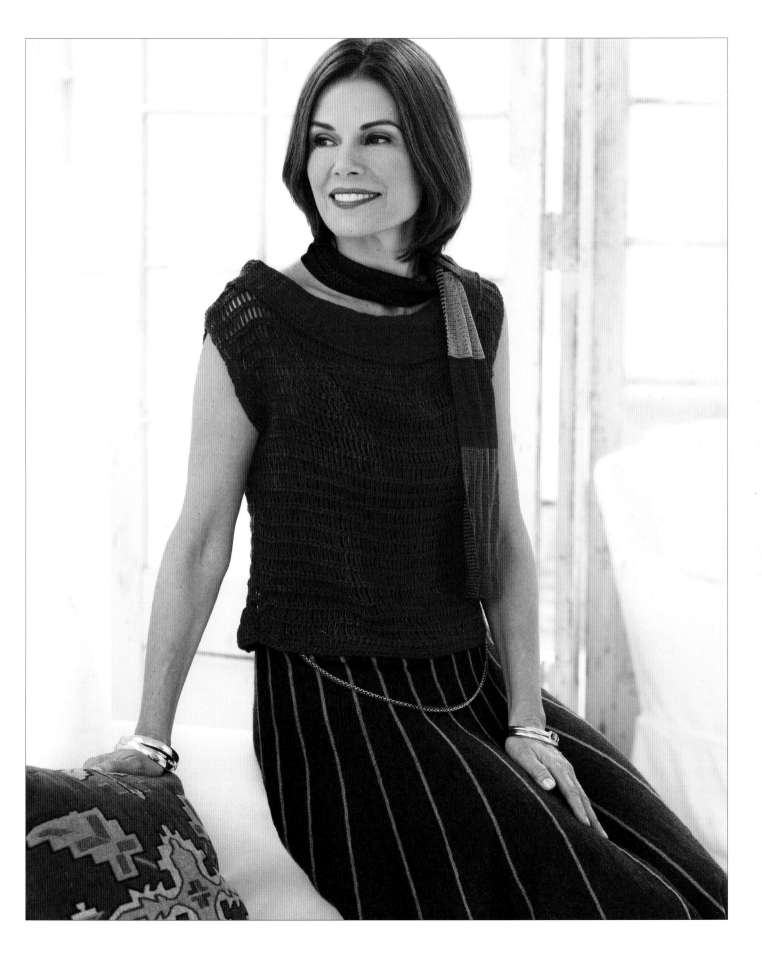

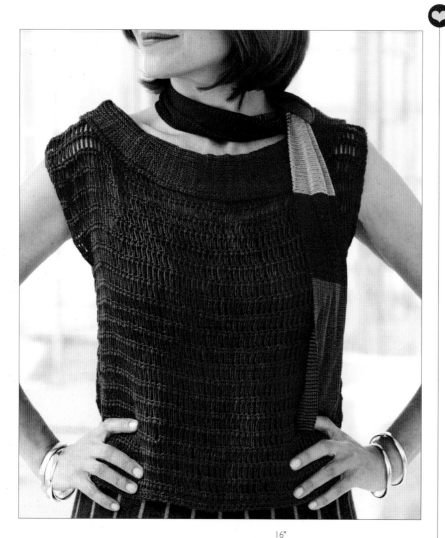

NOTE

1) Shell is worked in two pieces
and seamed up the sides.
To lengthen or shorten, simply
work more or fewer rows to
desired length.
2) On return rows, yo and
draw through first lp, [yo and draw
through 2 lps] until 1 lp rem.

BACK AND FRONT

With larger hook, ch 70 (74, 78,
86, 94).
Foundation row (RS) Pull up a lp
in 2nd ch from hook and in each
ch across, return.
Next row Tdks in each st
across, return.
Rep last row until piece measures
16½ (17, 17, 18, 18)"/42 (43, 43,
45.5, 45.5)cm from beg.
Next row Inserting hook as for
Tks, sc in each st across, fasten off.

NECKLINE STRIPS
(MAKE 2)
With smaller hook, ch 12.
Rows 1–96 Tks in each st across,
return. Fasten off when row 96
is complete.
Rotate to work in ends of rows.
Sc in each row across, turn.
Next row Ch 1, sc2tog across,
fasten off.

ASSEMBLY

Center one strip on top edge
of back and sew in place. Repeat
for front. Sew ends of strips
together and sew shoulder
seams. Sew side seams from hem
up, leaving 9"/22.9cm open for
each armhole.

FINISHING
EDGING
Rnd 1 Join yarn at bottom of side
seam. Ch 1, sc in each st of
foundation chain around, sl st to
join—138 (146, 154, 170, 186) sc.
Rnd 2 Ch 2, hdc in each st
around, sl st in top of ch-2 to
join, fasten off.
Block lightly to measurements. ♥

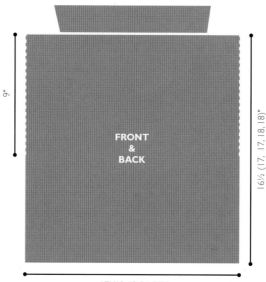

16"

9"

FRONT
&
BACK

16½ (17, 17, 18, 18)"

17 (18, 19, 21, 23)"

Hooded Scarf

Clever stitch combinations and a pretty edging all around give this soft hooded scarfette lovely drape and textural interest.

■■▢▭

SIZE
Instructions are written for one size.

MEASUREMENTS
LENGTH ALONG
BOTTOM EDGE
49"/124.5cm
HOOD DEPTH
9¾"/25cm
HOOD HEIGHT
10½"/26.5cm

MATERIALS
• 1 4oz/113g hank (each approx 440yd/402m) of Drew Emborsky *Gemstones* (superwash merino/nylon) in ruby ②
• Size H/8 (5mm) crochet hook *or size to obtain gauge*
• Stitch marker
• Tapestry needle

GAUGE
16 sts and 14 rows = 4"/10cm over hdc-blo using size H/8 (5mm) crochet hook.
➤ Take time to check gauge.

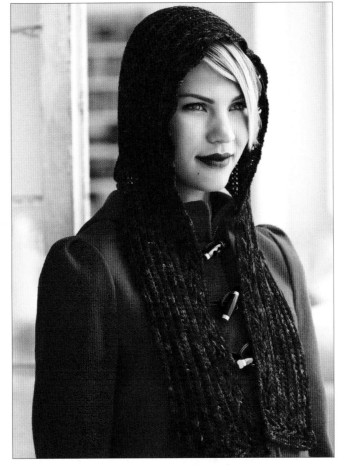

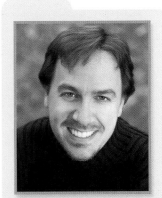

DREW'S STORY
Many of you know Drew Emborsky by another name: the Crochet Dude! Drew not only has a fantastic website full of tips and tricks of the crochet trade, but has also produced nine books, a line of yarns, and hooks and accessories from Boye. He's been crocheting since he was five—his mother taught him one snowed-in winter at Lake Tahoe, where he grew up, and the craft quickly became an obsession. His father, a World War II vet, was also an artist and crocheter, and Drew's parents raised a brood of crafty children. Drew has friends and family members who have been affected by heart disease. He loves to cook and experiment with new heart-healthy recipes: grilled wild salmon is a favorite, and his two cats, Chandler and Cleopatra, love it! His design was inspired by his sister-in-law Brenda, a survivor of heart disease.

NOTES
1) The scarf is worked first, then the hood. Finish by edging the entire project.
2) Ch-1 does *not* count as 1 hdc.
3) Ch-2 counts as 1 dc.

STITCH GLOSSARY
Dc-blo Double crochet in back loop only.
Hdc-blo Half double crochet in back loop only.
Sc-blo Single crochet in back loop only.

SCARF
Row 1 Ch 187, hdc into 2nd ch from hook and into each ch across—186 hdc.
Row 2 (RS) Ch 1, turn (does *not* count as first st), hdc-blo in each st to end.

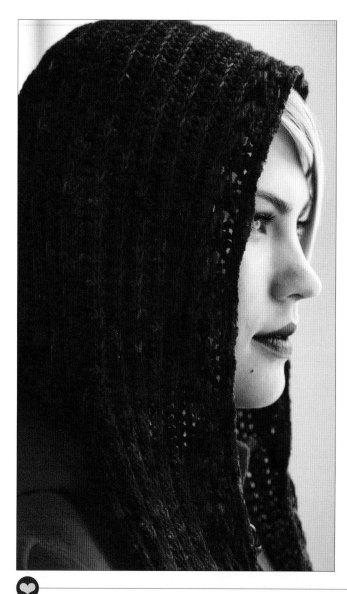

Rows 3–13 Rep row 2.

Row 14 Ch 2, turn (counts as first dc here and throughout), *sk 1 hdc, dc-blo in each of next 3 hdc, working in front of the sts just made, dc-blo in skipped hdc, inserting hook from back to front; rep from * to end, dc-blo in last st.

Row 15 Ch 2, turn, *sk 1 st, dc in each of next 3 sts, working in back of sts just made, dc in skipped st, inserting hook from front to back; rep from * to end, dc in last st. Fasten off.

SCARF EDGING

Work on both ends of scarf as foll:

Row 1 Working in ends of rows, with WS facing, attach yarn with sc in outer corner, work 21 more sc evenly spaced along end of scarf—22 sc.

Row 2 Ch 2, turn, *sk 1 sc, dc-blo in each of next 3 sc, working in front of sts just made, dc-blo in skipped st, inserting hook from back to front; rep from * to end, dc-blo in last st.

Row 13 Ch 2, turn, *sk 1 st, dc in each of next 3 sts, working in back of sts just made, dc in skipped st, inserting hook from front to back; rep from * to end, dc in last st.

Row 14 Ch 1, turn, sc in each st to end. Fasten off.

HOOD

Row 1 With WS facing and working in bottom of foundation ch, sk 51 sts, join with a hdc in next st, hdc in each of next 84 sts—85 hdc.

Rows 2–4 Ch 1, turn, (does *not* count as first st here and throughout), hdc-blo in each hdc to end.

Row 5 Ch 1, turn, hdc-blo in each of next 43 sts, place marker (pm) in top of st just made, hdc-blo to end.

Rows 6–16 Ch 1, turn, hdc-blo in each st until 2 sts rem before marker, hdc2tog, hdc in next st, pm in top of st just made, hdc2tog, hdc to end—83 hdc at end of row 6; 63 hdc at end of row 16.
Fasten off.

FINISHING

Fold hood in half at marker with RS facing. Whipstitch to seam back of hood, working through front lps of top of row 15 to maintain st pattern on RS.

EDGING

With RS facing, attach yarn with a sc-blo in any st along scarf area, sc-blo in each st around, and in each end of row along back edge of hood, working [sc, ch 1, sc] in each corner of scarf. Join rnd with sl st to first sc, fasten off. ❤

♥ DREW'S TIP
DREW MAKES SURE TO GET PLENTY OF EXERCISE by hiking in the mountains. Being in nature is also a great way to relieve stress!

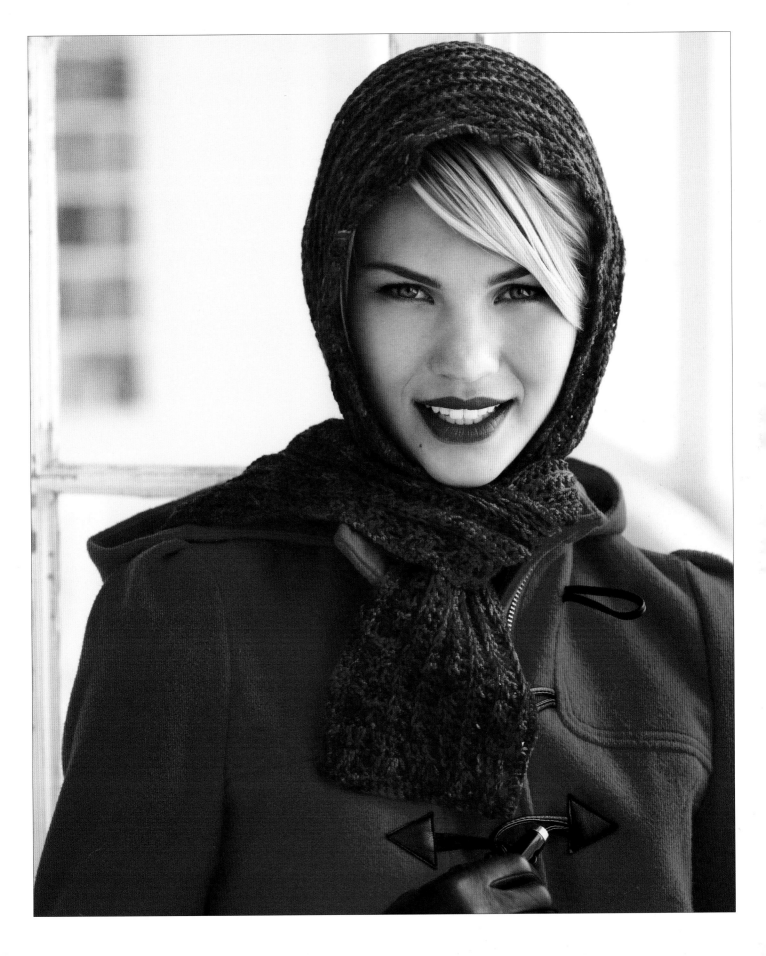

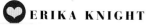 **ERIKA KNIGHT**

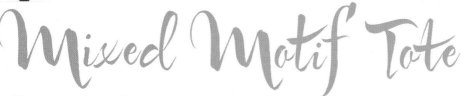
Mixed Motif Tote

Flaunt your skills with a bag that features favorite crochet motifs joined in an abstract pattern, with a contrasting felt lining peeking through.

MEASUREMENTS
WIDTH 17½"/44.5cm
HEIGHT 17"/43cm

MATERIALS
- 5 3½oz/100g hanks (each approx 87yd/80m) of Erika Knight *Maxi Wool* (wool) in #30 marni (6)
- Size M/13 (9mm) crochet hook *or size to obtain gauge*
- ½ yd/0.5m square heavyweight felt in contrasting color for lining
- Tapestry needle
- Large sheet of dressmaker's pattern paper or brown paper
- Pair of handles, 29"/73.5cm end to end

GAUGES
Eastern star motif = 8½"/21.5cm diameter using size M/13 (9mm) crochet hook.
Cluster circle motif = 5½"/14cm diameter using size M/13 (9mm) crochet hook.
Popcorn wheel square motif = 5½"/14cm square using size M/13 (9mm) crochet hook.
Shell cluster motif = 3¼"/8.5 cm diameter using size M/13 (9mm) crochet hook.
➤ Take time to check gauges.

STITCH GLOSSARY
Popcorn 5 dc in indicated st or sp, remove hook from working lp and insert in first of 5 dc just made, insert hook back in working lp and draw through dc, ch 1.
Sc2tog (single crochet 2 together) Pull up a lp in each of 2 indicated sts, yo and draw through all 3 lps on hook.
Dc2tog (double crochet 2 together) [Yo and pull up a lp in indicated st or sp, yo and draw through 2 lps] twice, yo and draw through all 3 lps on hook.
Dc3tog (double crochet 2 together) [Yo and pull up a lp in indicated st or sp, yo and draw through 2 lps] 3 times, yo and draw through all 4 lps on hook.

EASTERN STAR MOTIF (MAKE 6)
Ch 6, sl st in first ch forming a ring.
Rnd 1 ch 1, [sc in ring, ch 3] 12 times, sl st in first sc.
Rnd 2 Sl st in each of next 2 ch, ch 1, sc in same ch-3 sp, [ch 3, sc in next ch-3 sp] 11 times, ch 1, hdc in first sc.
Rnd 3 *Ch 6, sc in next ch-3 sp**, ch 3, sc in next ch-3 sp; rep from * 4 times more and from * to ** once more, ch 1, dc in hdc.
Rnd 4 *[5 dc, ch 2, 5 dc] in next ch-6 sp, **sc in next ch-3 sp; rep from * 4 times more and from * to ** once more, sc in dc. Fasten off.

CLUSTER CIRCLE MOTIF (MAKE 5)
Ch 6, sl st in first ch, forming a ring.
Rnd 1 Ch 3, dc2tog in ring, [ch 3, dc3tog in ring] 5 times, ch 1, hdc in first dc2tog.
Rnd 2 Ch 3, dc2tog in sp formed by hdc, *[ch 3, dc3tog] twice in next sp, rep from * 4 times more, ch 3, dc3tog in last sp, ch 1, hdc in first dc2tog. Fasten off.

POPCORN WHEEL SQUARE MOTIF (MAKE 4)
Ch 6, sl st in first ch, forming a ring.
Rnd 1 Ch 3 (counts as 1 dc), popcorn in ring counting beg ch-3 as first dc of popcorn, [ch 3, popcorn in ring] 7 times, ch 3, sl st in first popcorn.
Rnd 2 Ch 3 (counts as 1 dc), 2 dc in next ch-3 sp, [9 dc in next sp, 2 dc in next sp] 3 times, 8 dc in last sp, sl st in top of beg ch 3. Fasten off.

SHELL CLUSTER MOTIF (MAKE 14)
Ch 4, sl st in first ch, forming a ring.
Rnd 1 *Ch 3, 3 dc in ring, ch 3, sl st in ring (petal made), rep from * 3 times more. Fasten off.

BASE
Ch 9.
Row 1 Sc in 2nd ch from hook and in each ch across—8 sts.
Row 2 (inc) Ch 1, 2 sc in first sc, sc in each sc to last sc, 2 sc in last sc—10 sts.

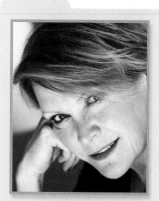

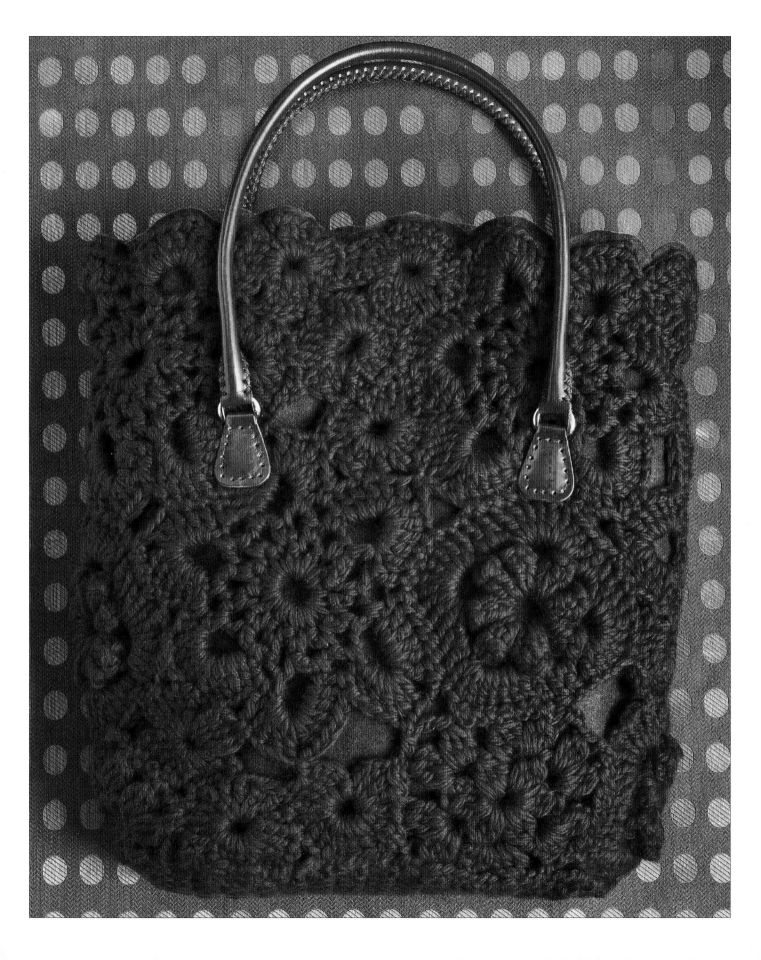

MOTIF 1: EASTERN STAR

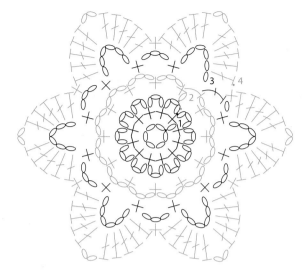

STITCH KEY

- • sl st
- ⬭ ch
- ✕ sc
- ⊤ hdc
- ⊤ dc
- ⬍ CL3
- ⬗ Popcorn

MOTIF 2: CLUSTER CIRCLE

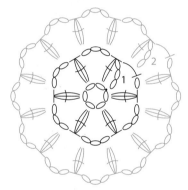

MOTIF 3: POPCORN WHEEL SQUARE

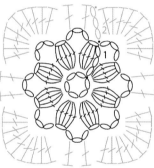

MOTIF 4: SHELL CLUSTER

SIDE 1 ASSEMBLY

SIDE 2 ASSEMBLY

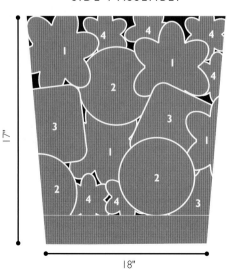

17"

18"

18"

Row 3 Rep row 2—12 sts.
Row 4 Ch 1, sc in each sc to end.
Rep row 4 until piece measures 10½"/26.5cm.
Next row (dec) Ch 1, sc2tog over first 2 sc, sc in each sc to last 2 sc, sc2tog over last 2 sc—10 sts.
Rep last row once more—8 sts.
Fasten off.

FINISHING

Block base and motifs lightly to measurements.
Make a paper pattern for the base of the felt lining by drawing around the crochet base, and adding a ½"/1.5cm seam allowance.
Draw a rectangle 35½"/90cm x 16½"/42cm on the sheet of dressmaker's paper.
Position the motifs, right side up, on top of the paper pattern as shown on assembly diagram and as close together as possible. Nudge the motifs into shapes that allow them to fit together tightly and touch their neighbors. Pin the motifs to the paper. Sew the motifs together with overcast stitches, leaving all motifs pinned to the paper until you have finished sewing them together. Remove pins and sew side seam. Pin and sew bag to base, easing in any extra fabric on body of bag.

LINING

Cut out a 36½"/92.5cm x 18"/45.5cm rectangle of felt, and sew short edges together to make a tube that will fit inside the bag.
Cut a felt base using the paper pattern you have drawn.
Pin and sew base to lining, easing in any extra fabric on body of bag. Insert lining into bag and pin it to motifs around top. Using matching thread, backstitch around top of bag through both layers. Cut away surplus felt from top of bag. Sew on handles. ❤

❤ CHARLES VOTH

Lace Swing Coat

Go for maximum drama with this long and loose coat, featuring a poinsettia lace pattern crocheted in a luxurious cashmere blend.

■■■◻

SIZES
Instructions are written for size X-Small. Changes for Small, Medium, Large, X-Large, and XX-Large are in parentheses. (Shown in size Small.)

MEASUREMENTS
BUST 38½ (42½, 45½, 50, 53½, 58½)"/97.5 (108, 115.5, 127, 136, 148.5)cm

MATERIALS
• 8 (8, 9, 9, 10, 10) 4oz/113g hanks (each approx 356yd/325m) of HandMaiden Fine Yarns *Casbah Sock* (wool/nylon/cashmere) in ruby ❶
• Size G/6 (4mm) crochet hook *or size to obtain gauge*
• Tapestry needle
• Stitch markers

GAUGES
2½ pat reps (47 sts on a RS row) = 6"/15cm and 9 rows = 4"/10cm unblocked using size G/6 (4mm) crochet hook.
2 pat reps (38 sts on a RS row) = 6"/15cm and 10 rows = 4"/10cm blocked using size G/6 (4mm) crochet hook.
➤ Take time to check gauges.

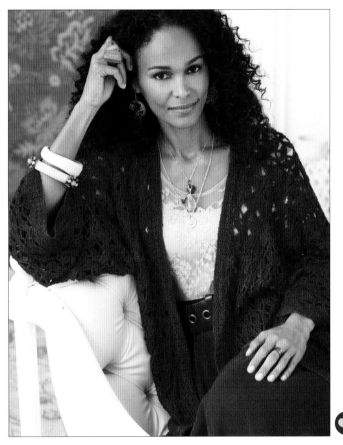

STITCH GLOSSARY
Str2tog (split treble 2 stitches together) Work tr in same st as last dc, leaving last 2 lps on hook, sk 8 sts, work 2nd tr in next st, closing last 3 lps on hook at one time, ch 3, dc in same st as last tr.

NOTES
1) Body is worked from center back to armholes, then out to front in one piece.
2) Ch-2 counts as 1 hdc.

POINSETTIA LACE PATTERN
One pat rep counts as 19 sts on a row 2 or 4.
Row 1 (WS) Ch 5, turn, sk 3 sts, (tr, ch 3, dc) in next st, ch 3, sk next 4 sts, *sc in next st, ch 3, sk 4 sts, dc in next st, ch 3, str2tog, ch 3, dc in same st as last tr; ch 3, sk 4 sts; rep from * to last 10 sts, sc in next st, ch 3, sk 4 sts, dc in next st, ch 3, tr in same st as last dc, leaving last 2 lps on hook, sk 4

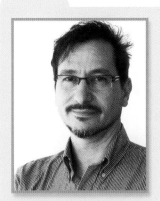

CHARLES'S STORY
A native of Cali, Colombia, Charles learned to crochet as a young boy from his mother and a friend of hers—and he's been hooked ever since. These days you can find him at home in Ontario, Canada, where he designs crochet and knitwear, creates and edits crochet diagrams and knitting charts, and spends his free time with his wife and their English cocker spaniel, Duncan. Charles has a close friend who underwent open-heart surgery and whose father and brother both suffer from Marfan's syndrome, which causes defects in the heart valves and aorta. And heart disease personally touched Charles when he lost his grandfather and two uncles to it—a perpetual reminder to care for his heart.

❤ **CHARLES'S TIP**
SINCE CHARLES HAS BEEN HIT SO CLOSE TO HOME BY HEART DISEASE, he's careful to mind his health by staying active (he loves to swim) and making healthy food choices. One of his favorite recipes is for gluten-free plötz, a traditional German fruit bar.

sts, dtr in last st, closing last 3 lps on hook at one time.

Row 2 (RS) Ch 1, turn, sc in first st, *[(sc, hdc, 2 dc) in next ch-3 sp, dc in next dc, (2 dc, hdc, sc) in next ch-3 sp] twice, sc in next st; rep from * across.

Row 3 (WS) Ch 1, turn, *sc in first st, ch 3, sk 4 sts, dc in next st, ch 3, str2tog, ch 3, dc in same st as last tr; ch 3, sk 4 sts; rep from * to last st, sc in last st.

Row 4 (RS) Ch 1, turn, *(sc, hdc, 2 dc) in next ch-3 sp, dc in next dc, (2 dc, hdc, sc) in next ch-3 sp, sc in next sc, (sc, hdc, 2 dc) in next ch-3 sp, dc in next dc, (2 dc, hdc, sc) in next ch-3 sp; rep from * across.

Rep rows 1–4 for poinsettia lace pat.

LEFT BODY

Ch 134 (134, 134, 146, 146, 146).

Row 1 (WS) Working into back/bump of starting ch across, sc in 2nd ch from hook, *ch 3, sk 3 ch, dc in next ch, ch 3, str2tog, ch 3, dc in same ch as last tr; ch 3, sk 3 ch, sc in next ch; rep from * across—11 (11, 11, 12, 12, 12) pat reps.

Row 2 (RS) Work row 4 of poinsettia lace pat across.

Rows 3–22 (24, 26, 28, 30, 32) Work rows 1–4 of poinsettia lace pat 5 (5, 6, 6, 7, 7) times, then rep rows 1–2 of pat 0 (1, 0, 1, 0, 1) time more.

LEFT ARMHOLE

Row 1 (WS) Ch 1, turn, sc in first st, sc in next sc, *sk 1 st, sc in each of next 2 sts; rep from * across—141 (141, 141, 153, 153, 153) sc.

Row 2 (RS) Ch 2 (counts as 1 hdc here and throughout), turn, (hdc, sc) in next st, *sk next st, (hdc, sc) in next st; rep from * to last st, hdc in last st.

Sizes X-Small, Small, and Medium only

Row 3 (WS) Ch 2, turn, *sk 1 hdc, (hdc, sc) in next sc; rep from * 44 times more, hdc in next hdc, leave rem sts unworked—90 sts.

Row 4 (RS) Ch 2, turn, *sk 1 hdc, (hdc, sc) in next sc; rep from * across, ending with hdc between last 2 sts.

Row 5 Rep row 4, but do not work last hdc, ch 52.

Row 6 Turn, working in back/bump of ch, (hdc, sc) in 3rd ch from hook, *sk 1 ch, (hdc, sc) in next ch; rep from * to first sc, (hdc, sc) in each sc across (sk each hdc), ending with hdc between last 2 sts.

Row 7 Ch 2, turn, (hdc, sc) in each sc across, ending with hdc in between last 2 sts.

Sizes Large (X-Large, XX-Large) only

Rows 3–4 (4, 6) Ch 2, turn, *sk 1 hdc, (hdc, sc) in next sc; rep from * across, ending with hdc between last 2 sts.

Row 5 (5, 7) (WS) Ch 2, turn, *sk 1 hdc, (hdc, sc) in next sc; rep from * 44 times more, hdc in next hdc, leave rem sts unworked—90 sts.

Row 6 (6, 8) (RS) Rep row 3.

Row 7 (7, 9) Rep row 4, but do not work last hdc and do not turn, ch 65.

Row 8 (8, 10) Working in back/bump of ch, (hdc, sc) in 3rd ch from hook, *sk 1 ch, (hdc, sc) in next ch; rep from * to first sc, (hdc, sc) in each sc across (sk each hdc), ending with hdc between last 2 sts.

Rows 9 (9, 11)–11 (11, 15) Ch 2, turn, (hdc, sc) in each sc across, ending with hdc between last 2 sts.

LEFT FRONT

Sizes X-Small (Medium, X-Large) only

Set-up row (RS) Ch 1, turn, *sc in next st, (sc, hdc) in next st, dc in next st, 2 dc in next st, dc in next st, (dc, hdc) in next st, sc in next st, (sc, hdc) in next st, dc in next st, 2 dc in next st, dc in next st, (dc, hdc) in next st, dc in next st, 2 dc in next st, dc in next st, hdc, 2 dc in next st, (hdc, dc) in next st, dc in next st, 2 dc in next st, dc in next st, (hdc, sc) in next st; rep from * across.

Row 1 Work row 3 of poinsettia lace pat.

Row 2 Work row 4 of poinsettia lace pat.

Rows 3–13 (17, 21) Work rows 1–4 of poinsettia lace pat 2 (3, 4) times, then rows 1–3 once more.

Sizes Small (Large, XX-Large) only

Set-up row (RS) Ch 1, turn, *(sc, hdc) in next st, dc in next st, 2 dc in next st, dc in next st, (dc, hdc) in next st, sc in next st, 2 sc in next st, hdc in next st, 2 dc in next st, dc in next st, 2 dc in next st, hdc, 2 dc in next st, (hdc, dc) in next st, dc in next st, 2 dc in next st, dc in next st, (hdc, sc) in next st, sc in next st, (sc, hdc) in next st, dc in next st, 2 dc in next st, dc in next st, (dc, hdc) in next st, sc in next st; rep from * across.

Rows 1–15 (19, 23) Work rows 1–4 of poinsettia lace pat 3 (4, 5) times, then rows 1–3 once.

LEFT NECKLINE

Row 1 (RS) Ch 1, 4 sc in first ch-sp, sc in next dc, 4 sc in next ch-sp, sc in next st, (2 sc, 1 hdc) in next ch-sp, dc in next dc, cont in poinsettia lace pat (row 4) for 33 more sts, place stitch marker in st just made (a sc), cont in established pat across—13 sc, 2 hdc, 3 dc, and 10 (10, 10, 11, 11, 11) pat reps.

Row 2 Ch 5, turn, work in poinsettia lace pat (row 1) to stitch marker, sc in marked st, ch 3, sk 4 sts, dc in next st, ch 3, dc in same dc just worked but leave last 2 lps on hook, sk 8 sts, dc in next st closing last 3 lps on hook at once, ch 3, dc in same st as last dc, ch 3, sk 4 sts, sc in next sc, ch 4, sk 4 sts, sc in next dc, sk 8, tr in next dc—8½ (8½, 8½, 9½, 9½, 9½) pat reps, 5 ch-sps, 1 tr.

Row 3 Ch 1, turn, 4 sc in first ch-sp, sc in next sc, 3 sc in next ch-sp, sc in next st, 3 sc in next ch-sp, sc in next dc, (hdc, dc, hdc, sc) in next ch-sp, (sc, hdc, 2dc) in next ch-sp, dc in next dc, (2 hdc, 2 sc) in next ch-sp, sc in next st, cont in poinsettia lace pat (row 2) across next 19 sts, place marker (pm) in st just made, cont in pat across—20 sc, 5 hdc, 4 dc, and 8 (8, 8, 9, 9, 9) pat reps.

Row 4 Ch 1, turn, work in poinsettia lace pat (row 3) to stitch marker, ch 3, sk 4 sts, (dc, ch 1, dc) in next st, ch 1, sk 8 sts, (dc, ch 1, dc) in next st, sk 4 sts, tr in next sc—20 sc, 9 hdc, 9 dc, and 6½ (6½, 6½, 7½, 7½, 7½) pat reps.

Row 5 Ch 1, turn, (sc in next ch-sp, sc in next dc) twice, 2 sc in next ch-sp, sc in next dc, (sc, 2 hdc, sc) in next ch-sp, (sc, 3 hdc) in next ch-sp, sc in next dc, 3 sc in next ch-sp, sc in next st, (2 sc, hdc, dc) in next ch-sp, work in poinsettia lace pat (row 4) for 15 more sts, pm in st just made, cont in pat across—5 sc and 6½ (6½, 6½, 7½, 7½, 7½) pat reps.

Row 6 Ch 5, turn, work in poinsettia lace pat (row 1) to marker; move marker up one row, ch 2, sk 4 sts, (dc, ch 1, dc) in next dc, ch 1, sk 7 sts, dc2tog—3 ch-sps, 4 dc, 6½ (6½, 6½, 7½, 7½, 7½) pat reps.

Row 7 Ch 1, turn, sc in next dc, sc in next ch-sp, sc in next dc, 2sc in next ch-2 sp, cont in pat across—5 sc and 6½ (6½, 6½, 7½, 7½, 7½) reps.

Row 8 Ch 1, turn, *sc in each of next 2 sts, sk 1 st; rep from * to marker, then work 68 sc evenly across neckline. Fasten off.

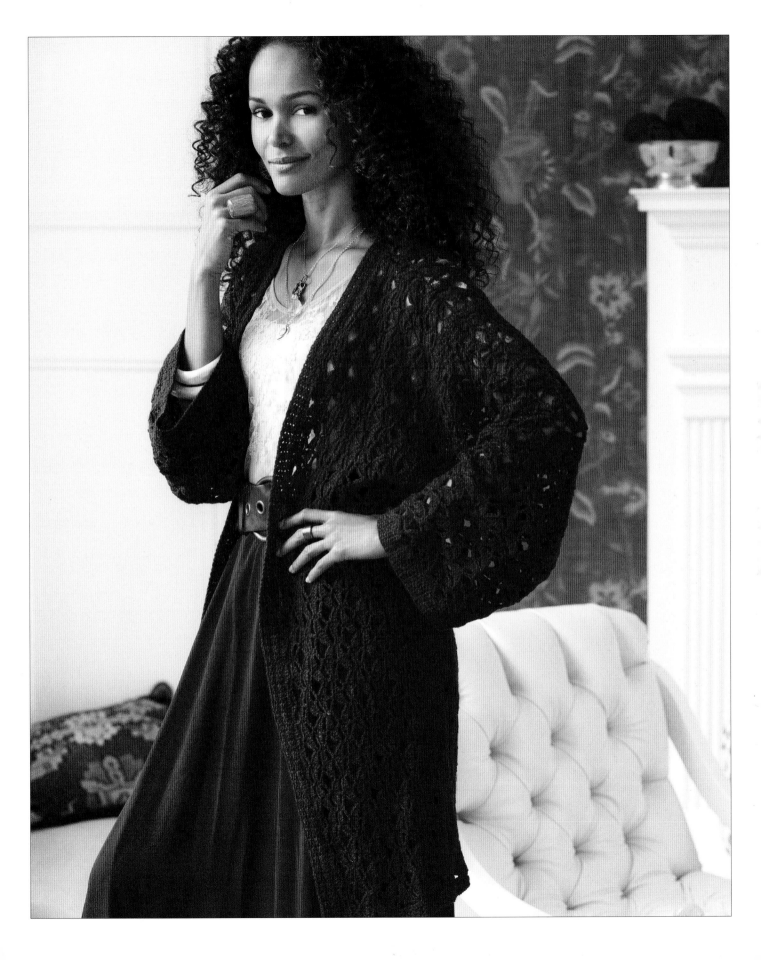

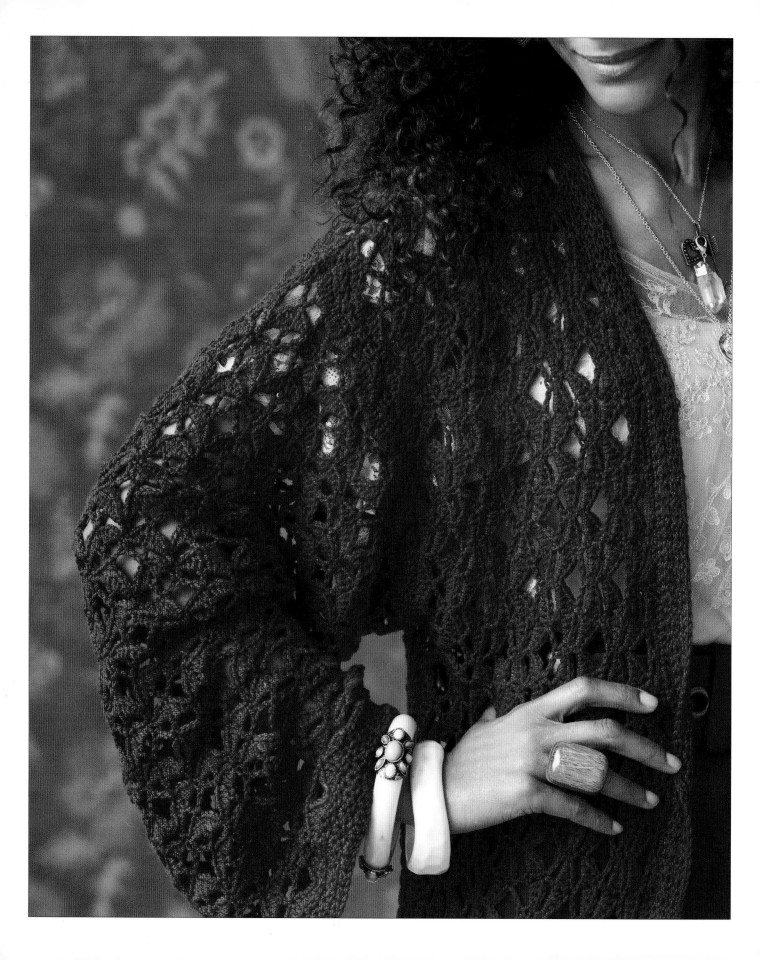

RIGHT BODY

With WS of left body facing, sl st to join in opposite side of first ch.

Row 1 (WS) Working into both lps of ch sts used on left body, *ch 3, sk 3 ch, dc in next ch, ch 3, str2tog, ch 3, dc in same ch as last tr, ch 3, sk 3 ch, sc in next ch; rep from * across—11 (11, 11, 12, 12, 12) pat reps in mirror image to row 1 of left body.

Row 2 (RS) Ch 1, turn, work row 4 of poinsettia lace pat.

Rows 3–22 (24, 26, 28, 30, 32) Work rows 1–4 of poinsettia lace pat 5 (5, 6, 6, 7, 7) times, then rep rows 1–2 of pat 0 (1, 0, 1, 0, 1) time more.

RIGHT ARMHOLE

Rows 1 and 2 Work as for left armhole.

Row 3 (WS) Ch 2, turn, *sk 1 hdc, (hdc, sc) in next sc; rep from * across, hdc in last st.

Sizes X-Small, Small, and Medium only

Row 4 (RS) Ch 2, turn, *sk 1 hdc, (hdc, sc) in next sc; rep from * 44 times more, hdc in next hdc, leave rem sts unworked—90 sts.

Row 5 (WS) Ch 2, turn, *sk 1 hdc, (hdc, sc) in next sc; rep from * across, ending with hdc between last 2 sts.

Row 6 Rep row 4, do not work last hdc and do not turn, ch 52.

Row 7 Turn, working in back/bump of ch, (hdc, sc) in 3rd ch from hook, *sk 1 ch, (hdc, sc) in next ch; rep from * to first sc, (hdc, sc) in each sc across (sk hdcs), ending with hdc between last 2 sts.

Rows 8 and 9 Ch 2, turn, (hdc, sc) in each sc across (sk hdcs), ending with hdc between last 2 sts.

Sizes Large (X-Large, XX-Large) only

Rows 4–5 (5, 7) Ch 2, *sk 1 hdc, (hdc, sc) in next sc; rep from * across, ending with hdc between last 2 sts.

Row 6 (6, 8) (RS) Ch 2, *sk 1 hdc, (hdc, sc) in next sc; rep from * 44 times more, hdc in next hdc, leave rem sts unworked—90 sts.

Row 7 (7, 9) (WS) Rep row 4.

Row 8 (8, 10) Rep row 4, do not work last hdc and do not turn, ch 65.

Row 9 (9, 11) Turn, working in back/bump of ch, (hdc, sc) in 3rd ch from hook, *sk 1 ch, (hdc, sc) in next ch; rep from * to first sc, (hdc, sc) in each sc across (sk hdcs), ending with hdc between last 2 sts.

Rows 10 (10, 12)–11 (11, 15) Rep row 4.

RIGHT FRONT

Sizes X-Small (Medium, X-Large) only

Set-up row (RS) Ch 1, turn, *sc in next st, (sc, hdc) in next st, dc in next st, 2 dc in next st, dc in next st, (dc, hdc) in next st, sc in next st, (sc, hdc) in next st, dc in next st, 2 dc in next st, dc in next st, (dc, hdc) in next st, sc in next st, 2 sc in next st, hdc in next st, 2 dc in next st, dc in next st, 2 dc in next st, (hdc, 2 sc) in next st, (hdc, dc) in next st, dc in next st, 2 dc in next st, dc in next st, (hdc, sc) in next st; rep from * across.

Row 1 Work row 3 of poinsettia lace pat.

Row 2 Work row 4 of poinsettia lace pat.

Rows 3–13 (17, 21) Work rows 1–4 of poinsettia lace pat 2 (3, 4) times, then rows 1–3 once.

Sizes S, (L, 2X) only

Set up row (RS) Ch 1, turn, *(sc, hdc) in next st, dc in next st, 2 dc in next st, dc in next st, (dc, hdc) in next st, sc in next st, 2 sc in next st, hdc in next st, 2 dc in next st, dc in next st, 2 dc in next st, hdc, 2 sc in next st, (hdc, dc) in next st, dc in next st, 2 dc in next st, dc in next st, (hdc, sc) in next st, sc in next st, (sc, hdc) in next st, dc in next st, 2 dc in next st, dc in next st, (hdc, sc) in next st, sc in next st, (sc, hdc) in next st, dc in next st, 2 dc in next st, dc in next st, (dc, hdc) in next st, sc in next st; rep from * across.

Rows 1–15 (19, 23) Work rows 1–4 of poinsettia lace pat 3 (4, 5) times, then rows 1–3 once.

RIGHT NECKLINE

With WS facing, counting in from beg of row 13 (15, 17, 19, 21, 23), sk (ch-3 sp, dc, ch-3 sp, str2tog, ch-3 sp), pm in next st. Turn.

Row 1 (RS) Work in poinsettia lace pat (row 4) to marker, (2 hdc, 2 sc) in next ch-3 sp, sc in next st—10¾ (10¾, 10¾, 11¾, 11¾, 11¾) pat reps, 2 hdc, 3 sc.

Row 2 Ch 1, turn, sk first sc, sl st in each of next 4 sts, ch 3, sk 8 sts, sc in next st, ch 3, sc in next st, ch 3, sk 4 sts, (hdc, ch 1, dc) in next dc, ch 1, sk 8 sts, (dc, ch 1, dc) in next dc, cont in poinsettia lace pat (row 1) to next str2tog made, pm in that st, cont in pat across—4 sl st, 7 ch-sps, 9 (9, 9, 10, 10, 10) pat reps.

Row 3 Work in poinsettia lace pat (row 2) to marker, sc in marked st, (2 sc, 2 hdc) in next ch-3 sp, dc in next dc, (2 dc, hdc, sc) in next ch-3 sp, (sc, 2 hdc) in next ch-sp, dc2tog across next ch and next st—8½ (8½, 8½, 9½, 9½, 9½) pat reps, 6 sc, 5 hdc, 3 dc, 1 dc2tog.

Row 4 Ch 3, turn, sk 7 sts, sl st in each of next 8 sts, ch 2, sk 2 sts, (hdc, ch 1, dc) in next dc, ch 2, sk 8 sts, (dc, ch 1, dc) in next dc, ch 3, sk 4 sts, sc in next sc, cont in poinsettia lace pat (row 3) to next sc, mark this sc, cont in pat across—6 ch-sps, 8 sl-sts, 7½ (7½, 7½, 8½, 8½, 8½) pat reps.

Row 5 Ch 1, turn, work in poinsettia lace pat (row 4) to marker, (sc, hdc, 2 dc) in next ch-3 sp, dc in next dc, (dc, hdc, 2 sc) in next ch-3 sp, sc in next st, 4 sc in next ch-3 sp, sc in next dc, (3 hdc, sc) in next ch-3 sp, (sc, hdc, sc) in next ch-3 sp—6½, (6½, 6½, 7½, 7½, 7½) pat reps, 12 sc, 6 hdc, 4 dc.

Row 6 Ch 1, turn, sk 1 st, sl st in each of next 14 sts, ch 1, sk 1 st, (hdc, ch 1, dc) in next dc, ch 1, sk 8 sts, (dc, ch 1, dc) in next dc, ch 3, sk 4 sts, sc in next sc, pm in sc just made, cont in poinsettia lace pat (row 1) across—14 sl-sts, 4 ch-sps, 6 (6, 6, 7, 7, 7) pat reps.

Row 7 Ch 1, turn, work in poinsettia lace pat (row 2) to marker, fasten off, leaving marker in place.

Row 8 With WS facing, sl st to join yarn at outer edge and work 68 sc evenly spaced across neck opening to marker, sc in each of next 2 sts, *sk 1 st, sc in each of next 2 sts; rep from * across. Fasten off.

SLEEVES (MAKE 2)
CUFF

Ch 83 (83, 83, 109, 109, 109).

Row 1 Working in back/bump of ch, sc in 2nd ch from hook and in each ch across—82 (82, 82, 108, 108, 108) sc.

Row 2 Ch 2, turn, *sk 1 st, (hdc, sc) in next st; rep from * across.

Rows 3–4 (4, 4, 6, 8, 10) Ch 2, turn, (hdc, sc) in each sc across (sk each hdc).

BODY OF SLEEVE

Row 1 (RS) Ch 1, turn, sc in each of next 3 sts, *[hdc in next st, 2 dc in next st, dc in next st, 2 dc in next st, hdc in next st], 2 sc in next st, rep between [ ], sc in next st, 2 sc in next st; rep from * across, sc in last st—6 (6, 6, 8, 8, 8) pat reps and 4 sc.

Row 2 (WS) Ch 5, sc in 3rd sc, cont in poinsettia lace pat (row 3) across, ending with ch 2, dc in last st.

Row 3 Ch 3, turn, (2 dc, sc) in ch-2 sp, cont in poinsettia lace pat (row 4) across, ending with (sc, hdc, 3 dc) in last ch-5 sp.

Row 4 Ch 6, str2tog with first tr going into base of ch, sk 8 sts, 2nd tr going into next dc, ch 3, dc into same st as tr, ch 3, sk 4 sts, sc in next sc, cont in poinsettia lace pat (row 1) across, ending with ch 3, dc in same st as tr.

Row 5 Ch 3, turn, (2 dc, hdc, sc) in first ch-sp, cont in poinsettia lace pat (row 2) across, ending with (sc, hdc, 2 dc) in last ch-sp, dc in last dc.

Row 6 Ch 5, turn, dc in base of t-ch, ch 3, cont in poinsettia lace pat (row 3) across, ending with (dc, ch 2, dc) in last st.

Row 7 Ch 2, turn, 2 dc in ch-sp, dc in next dc, (2 dc, hdc, sc) in next ch-sp, cont in poinsettia lace pat (row 4) across, ending with (2 dc, hdc) in last ch-5 sp.

Row 8 Ch 2, turn, sk 3 sts, dc in next st, ch 3, cont in poinsettia lace pat (row 1) across, ending with ch 2, sl st in last st.

Row 9 Ch 3, turn, dc in ch-sp, dc in next dc, cont in poinsettia lace pat (row 2) across, ending with 2 dc between last 2 sts.

Row 10 Ch 4, (tr, ch 3, dc) in 3rd st, ch 3, sk 4 sts, sc in next sc, cont in poinsettia lace pat (row 3) across, ending with tr2tog with 2nd tr going in last st.

Row 11 Ch 1, turn, sc in str2tog, cont in poinsettia lace pat (row 4) across, ending with sc in top ch of t-ch.

Row 12 Ch 6, turn, str2tog with first tr in base of ch, sk 6 sts, 2nd tr in next dc, ch 3, dc in same st as last tr, ch 3, sk 4 sts, sc in next sc, cont in poinsettia lace pat (row 1) across, ending with 2nd tr of last str2tog in last st, ch 2, tr in last st.

Row 13 Ch 3, turn, (hdc, sc) in ch-2 sp, sc in str2tog, cont in poinsettia lace pat (row 2) across, ending with (sc, hdc, tr) in last ch-sp.

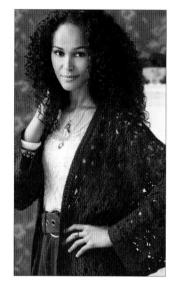

Row 14 Ch 5, turn, sk (tr, hdc), sc in next sc, cont in poinsettia lace pat across, ending with ch 2, dc in last st.

Rep rows 3–14 until there are an even 8 (8, 8, 10, 10, 10) pat reps across—153 (153, 153, 191, 191, 191) sts on a pat row 4—then cont to work even in poinsettia lace pat until sleeve measures 16½ (16½, 16½, 17, 17½, 18)"/42 (42, 42, 43, 44.5, 45.5)cm from start. Fasten off.

FINISHING
Block pieces lightly to measurements. Sew shoulder seams.

EDGING
Set-up rnd With WS facing, sl st to join at center back, ch 1, sc evenly across toward front corner, work 3 sc in corner, (hdc, sc) in every other st up front edge and neckline to 1 st before shoulder seam, sc2tog in last st of neckline and first st of back neck, sc an even number of sts evenly across back neck to shoulder seam, sc2tog in last st of back neck and first st of other front edge, (hdc, sc) in every other st along other neckline and front edge to bottom corner, work 3 sc in corner, sc evenly across to

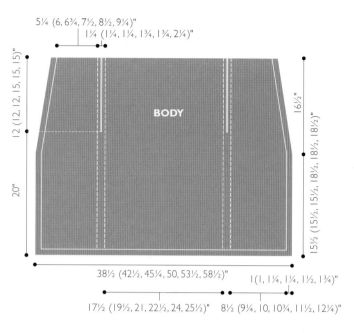

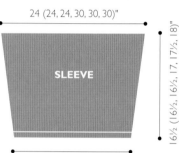

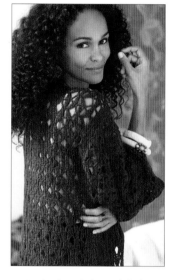

center back and sl st to join in first ch, turn, pm in center sc in each corner.

Rnd 1 (RS) Ch 1, (hdc, sc) in every other st to corner, 3 hdc in marked corner st, move marker to center st of 3 sts just made, (hdc, sc) in each sc (sk hdc) to back neck, (hdc, sc) in every other st to opposite front edge, (hdc, sc) in each sc (sk hdc) to corner, 3 hdc in marked corner st, move marker to center st of 3 sts just made, (hdc, sc) in every

other st to center back, sl st to ch 1 to join rnd.

Row 2 (WS) Ch 1, turn, (hdc, sc) in each sc (sk hdc) around, working 3 hdc in each marked corner and moving marker to center hdc, sl st to ch 1 to join rnd.

Rows 3–4 (4, 4, 6, 8, 10) Rep row 2. Fasten off.

Sew sleeves into armhole openings and sew sleeve seams. Block lightly to measurements. ❤

Body schematic labels:
5¼ (6, 6¾, 7½, 8½, 9¼)"
1¼ (1¼, 1¼, 1¾, 1¾, 2¼)"
BODY
16½"
12 (12, 12, 15, 15, 15)"
20"
15½ (15½, 15½, 18½, 18½, 18½)"
38½ (42½, 45¼, 50, 53½, 58½)"
1 (1, 1¼, 1¼, 1½, 1¾)"
17½ (19½, 21, 22½, 24, 25½)"
8½ (9¼, 10, 10¾, 11½, 12¼)"

Sleeve schematic labels:
24 (24, 24, 30, 30, 30)"
SLEEVE
16½ (16½, 16½, 17, 17½, 18)"
19½ (19½, 19½, 25½, 25½, 25½)"

Asymmetrical Sweater

An asymmetrical shape and side-to-side construction are the elements of a versatile and modern design that shows a little shoulder.

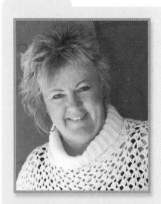

■ ■ ■ ▬

SIZES
Instructions are written for size X-Small. Changes for Small, Medium, Large, and X-Large are in parentheses. (Shown in size Medium.)

MEASUREMENTS
WIDTH (FROM CUFF TO CUFF, EXCLUDING CUFFS) 40¾ (41¾, 43, 44¼, 45¼)"/103.5 (106, 109, 112.5, 115)cm
HIPS 33½ (35½, 38, 40½, 42½)"/85 (90, 96.5, 103, 108)cm
LENGTH FROM CENTER NECK 22"/56cm

MATERIALS
• 8 (8, 9, 10, 11) 1¾oz/50g balls (each approx 110yd/100m) of Noro *Silk Garden* (silk/mohair/lambswool) in #84 reds (④)
• Size G/6 (4mm) crochet hook *or size to obtain gauge*
• Stitch markers
• Tapestry needle

GAUGE
18 sts and 7 rows = 4"/10cm over pattern st using size F/5 (3.75mm) crochet hook.
➤Take time to check gauge.

STITCH GLOSSARY
dc2tog (double crochet 2 together) *Yo, insert hook in indicated st and draw up a loop, yo and draw through 2 loops on

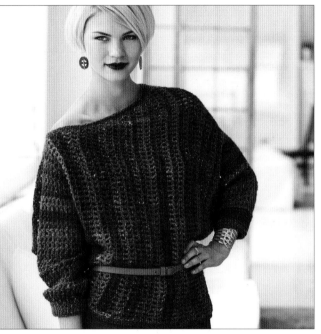

hook; rep from * once more in next indicated st (sk ch-1 sp), yo and draw through all 3 loops on hook.
FPdc (front post double crochet) Yo, insert hook from front to back to front around post of indicated st, draw up a loop, [yo and draw through 2 loops on hook] twice.

NOTE
Sweater is worked sideways from cuff to cuff.

SLEEVE
Ch 64.
Row 1 (RS) Dc in 6th ch from hook (counts as dc, ch-1 sp), *ch 1, sk 1 ch, dc in next ch; rep from * to end—30 ch-1 sps.

Row 2 Ch 4 (counts as dc, ch-1 sp), turn, dc in first dc, *ch 1, sk ch-1 sp, dc in next dc; rep from * across to t-ch, ch 1, sk 1 ch on t-ch, dc in next ch of t-ch—31 ch-1 sps.
Rep row 2 eleven times more—42 ch-1 sps.
Row 14 Ch 4 (counts as dc, ch-1 sp), turn, dc in first dc, ch 1, sk next ch-1 sp, (dc, ch 1, dc) in next dc, *ch 1, sk next ch-1 sp, dc in next dc; rep from * across to t-ch, ch 1, (dc, ch 1, dc) in 3rd ch of t-ch—45 ch-1 sps.
Rep row 14 eleven times more—78 ch-1 sps.
Row 26 Rep row 2—79 ch-1 sps.

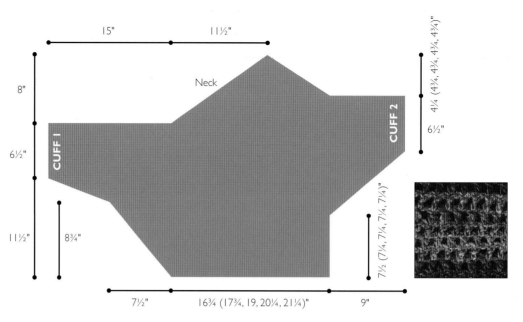

BACK

Row 1 Ch 4 (counts as dc, ch-1 sp), turn, sk first dc, sk next ch-1 sp, dc in next dc, *ch 1, sk ch-1 sp, dc in next dc; rep from * across for 39 sps total (including t-ch sp)—39 ch-1 sps.

Row 2 Ch 4 (counts as dc, ch-1 sp), turn, dc in first dc, *ch 1, sk ch-1 sp, dc in next dc; rep from * across to t-ch, ch 1, dc in 3rd ch of t-ch—40 ch-1 sps.

Row 3 Ch 4 (counts as dc, ch-1 sp), turn, sk first dc, sk next ch-1 sp, dc in next dc, *ch 1, sk next ch-1 sp, dc in next dc; rep from * across to t-ch, ch 1, (dc, ch 1, dc) in 3rd ch of t-ch—41 ch-1 sps. Rep rows 2 and 3 eight times more—57 ch-1 sps. Lay working yarn down.

FRONT

Row 1 Skip next ch-1 sp on row 26 from end of back row 1, join yarn with sl st to next dc, ch 4 (counts as dc, ch-1 sp), sk next ch-1 sp, dc in next dc, *ch 1, sk next ch-1 sp, dc in next dc; rep from * across to t-ch, ch 1, dc in 3rd ch of t-ch—39 ch-1 sps.

Row 2 Ch 4 (counts as dc, ch-1 sp), turn, sk first dc, sk next ch-1 sp, dc in next dc, *ch 1, sk next ch-1 sp, dc in next dc; rep from * across to t-ch, ch 1, (dc, ch 1, dc) in 3rd ch of t-ch—40 ch-1 sps.

Row 3 Ch 4 (counts as dc, ch-1 sp), turn, dc in first dc, *ch 1, sk ch-1 sp, dc in next dc; rep from * across to t-ch, ch 1, dc in 3rd ch of t-ch—41 ch-1 sps. Rep rows 2 and 3 eight times—57 ch-1 sps. Fasten off.

SHOULDER

Row 1 (joining row) Turn, pick up yarn at end of last row of back, ch 4 (counts as dc, ch-1 sp), sk first dc, sk next ch-1 sp, dc in next dc, *ch 1, sk next ch-1 sp, dc in next dc; rep from * across to t-ch, ch 1, dc in 3rd ch of t-ch, ch 1, place marker (pm) in ch-1 sp, dc in first dc of front panel, rep from * across to t-ch, ch 1, dc in 3rd ch of t-ch—115 ch-1 sps.

Row 2 Ch 4 (counts as dc, ch-1 sp), turn, sk first dc, sk next ch-1 sp, dc in next dc, *ch 1, sk next ch-1 sp, dc in next dc; rep from * across to dc before marker, dc2tog over next 2 dc (sk ch-1 sp between), move marker, rep from * across to t-ch, ch 1, dc in 3rd ch of t-ch—114 ch-1 sps.

Row 3 Ch 4 (counts as dc, ch-1 sp), turn, sk first dc, sk next ch-1 sp, dc in next dc, *ch 1, sk next ch-1 sp, dc in next dc; rep from * across to dc before marker, dc2tog over next 2 dc (sk ch-1 sp, dc2tog, ch-1 sp between), move marker, rep from * across to t-ch, ch 1, dc in 3rd ch of t-ch—112 ch-1 sps. Rep row 3 for 8 (10, 10, 10, 10) times more—96 (94, 94, 94, 94) ch-1 sps.

SIZES M, L, XL ONLY

Row 14 Ch 4 (counts as dc, ch-1 sp), turn, sk first dc, sk next ch-1 sp, dc in next dc, *ch 1, sk next ch-1 sp, dc in next dc; rep from * across to t-ch, ch 1, dc in 3rd ch of t-ch. Rep row 14 for 1 (3, 5) times more.

ALL SIZES

Fasten off.

OPPOSITE SLEEVE

Row 1 Turn, sk 17 (16, 16, 16, 16) ch-1 sps, join yarn to next dc with sl st, ch 2, dc2tog over prev and next dc, *ch 1, sk ch-1 sps, dc in next dc; rep from * 59 times total, ch 1, dc2tog over next 2 dc, leave remaining sts unworked—60 ch-1 sps.

Row 2 Ch 4 (counts as dc, ch-1 sp), turn, sk dc2tog, dc2tog over next 2 dc, *ch 1, sk next ch-1 sp, dc in next dc; rep from * across to last 2 dc, ch 1, dc2tog over last 2 dc—58 ch-1 sps.

Row 3 Ch 4 (counts as dc, ch-1 sp), turn, sk dc2tog, dc2tog over next 2 dc, *ch 1, sk next ch-1 sp, dc in next dc; rep from * across to dc2tog, ch 1, dc2tog over dc2tog and 3rd ch of t-ch—56 ch-1 sps. Rep row 3 thirteen times—30 ch-1 sps. Fasten off.

FINISHING

Block lightly to measurements. Fold sweater in half, matching underarm seams and bottom edges with RS facing. Whipstitch underarm seams together.

FIRST CUFF

With RS facing, join yarn with sl st to underarm seam at foundation chain.

Rnd 1 Ch 4 (counts as dc, ch-1 sp), [FPdc around next dc, ch 1] around, sl st to 3rd ch of t-ch.

Rnd 2 Ch 3 (counts as dc), do not turn, FPdc around each dc around, sl st to top of t-ch. Rep rnd 2 six times more, fasten off.

SECOND CUFF

With WS facing, join yarn with sl st to underarm seam at last row.

Rnd 1 Ch 4 (counts as dc, ch-1 sp), [FPdc around next dc, ch 1] around, sl st to 3rd ch of t-ch.

Rnd 2 Ch 3 (counts as dc), do not turn, FPdc around each dc around, sl st to top of t-ch. Rep rnd 2 six times, fasten off.

NECK EDGING

With RS facing, join yarn with sl st to back neck.

Rnd 1 Ch 1, sc evenly around neck, do *not* join.

Rnd 2 Turn, sc tbl in each sc around, do *not* join.

Rnd 3 Turn, sc tbl in each sc around, sl st to first sc, fasten off.

BOTTOM EDGING

Work as for neck edging around bottom edge.❤

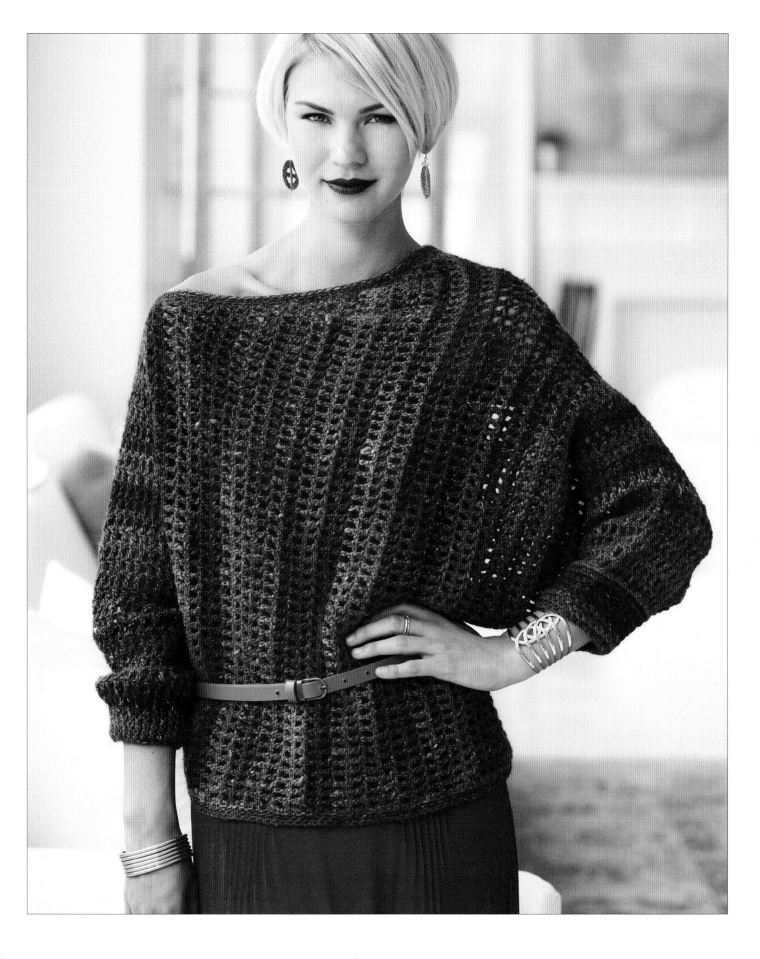

Textured Jacket

A crinkle stitch pattern in a subtly variegated yarn brings loads of texture to a structured jacket with a flattering fit.

SIZES
Instructions are written for size Small. Changes for sizes Medium, Large, X-Large, and XX-Large are in parentheses. (Shown in size Small.)

MEASUREMENTS
BUST (BUTTONED) 34½ (37½, 42½, 45, 50)"/87.5 (95, 108, 114, 127)cm
LENGTH 26 (26½, 27, 27½, 28)"/66 (67.5, 68.5, 70, 71)cm

MATERIALS
• 8 (9, 10, 11, 12) 3½oz/100g hanks (each approx 210yd/192m) of Malabrigo Yarn *Merino Worsted* (merino) in #611 Ravelry red (4)
• One each sizes K/10.5 and L/11 (6.5 and 8mm) crochet hook *or size to obtain gauge*
• 8 buttons, ⅞"/22mm diameter (shown: JHB International #32123)
• Tapestry needle

GAUGE
13 sts and 16 rows = 4"/10cm over crinkle st using size K/10.5 (6.5mm) crochet hook.
➤ Take time to check gauge.

CRINKLE STITCH
(over an even number of sts plus 1 for foundation ch)
Set-up row (RS) Sl st in 3rd ch from hook (beg ch-2 counts as first hdc), *hdc in next ch, sl st in next ch; rep from * across.
Row 1 Ch 2 (counts as hdc here and throughout), turn, sk first sl st, *sl st in next hdc, hdc in next sl st; rep from * across, sl st in top of turning ch.
Rep row 1 for crinkle st.

NOTES
1) Each hdc, sl st, and turning ch-2 counts as one st throughout.
2) To ensure random color distribution, work invisible stripes, alternating 2 rows from each of 2 skeins of yarn.
3) When instructed to work in crinkle st "as established," work a sl st in each hdc and an hdc in each sl st of previous row.

BACK
With smaller hook, ch 55 (61, 67, 73, 79).
Work crinkle st set-up row— 54 (60, 66, 72, 78) sts.
Work even in crinkle st until piece measures approx 18½"/47cm from beg, end with a WS row.

ARMHOLE SHAPING
Next row (RS) Turn, sl st in first 3 (5, 6, 7, 8) sts, work in crinkle st as established to last 2 (4, 5, 6, 7) sts; leave last 2 (4, 5, 6, 7) sts unworked—50 (52, 56, 60, 64) sts. **Note** First 2 (4, 5, 6, 7) sl sts of this row are not included in the st count. Do not work into these sts when working next row. Cont working in crinkle st as established AND dec 1 st at beg and end of every row 1 (1, 2, 0, 1) times. Then dec 1 st at beg and end of every other row 3 (3, 3, 4, 4) times—42 (44, 46, 52, 54) sts. **Note** To dec a st at beg of a row, sl st into the first st and then begin crinkle st in the 2nd st. To dec a st at end of a row, leave the last st unworked.
Work even in crinkle st until piece measures approx 26 (26½, 27, 27½, 28)"/66 (67.5, 68.5, 70, 71)cm from beg, end with a WS row. Fasten off.

LEFT FRONT
With smaller hook, ch 37 (39, 43, 45, 49).
Work crinkle st set-up row—36 (38, 42, 44, 48) sts.
Work even in crinkle st until piece measures approx 18½"/47cm from beg, end with a WS row.

ARMHOLE SHAPING
Next row (RS) Turn, sl st in first 3 (5, 6, 7, 8) sts, work in crinkle st as established to end—34 (34, 37, 38, 41) sts. **Note** First 2 (4, 5, 6, 7) sl sts of this row are not included in the st count. Do not work into these sts when working next row. Cont working in crinkle st as established AND dec 1 st at armhole edge every row 1 (1, 2, 0, 1) times. Then dec 1 st at armhole edge every other row 3 (3, 3, 4, 4) times—30 (30, 32, 34, 36) sts.

MELISSA'S STORY
One of the industry's most prolific designers, Melissa Leapman has fifteen books and more than seven hundred designs to her name. It's no wonder: she learned to crochet as a toddler (!) and hasn't stopped since. A denizen of fashion-forward New York City, Melissa has worked as a freelance designer for top names in fashion, and has appeared on television as an instructor. Despite not always having time to knit or crochet "for fun," she says she has the best job in the world—we agree! Melissa has known heart disease personally since childhood: her mother underwent open-heart surgery at only thirty-three. The family altered their way of life dramatically to accommodate her condition, and forty years later, Melissa is devoted to a vegetarian diet to maintain her heart health. Managing stress is also an important factor, and something Melissa pays special attention to, with deadlines always looming.

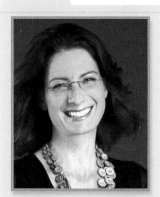

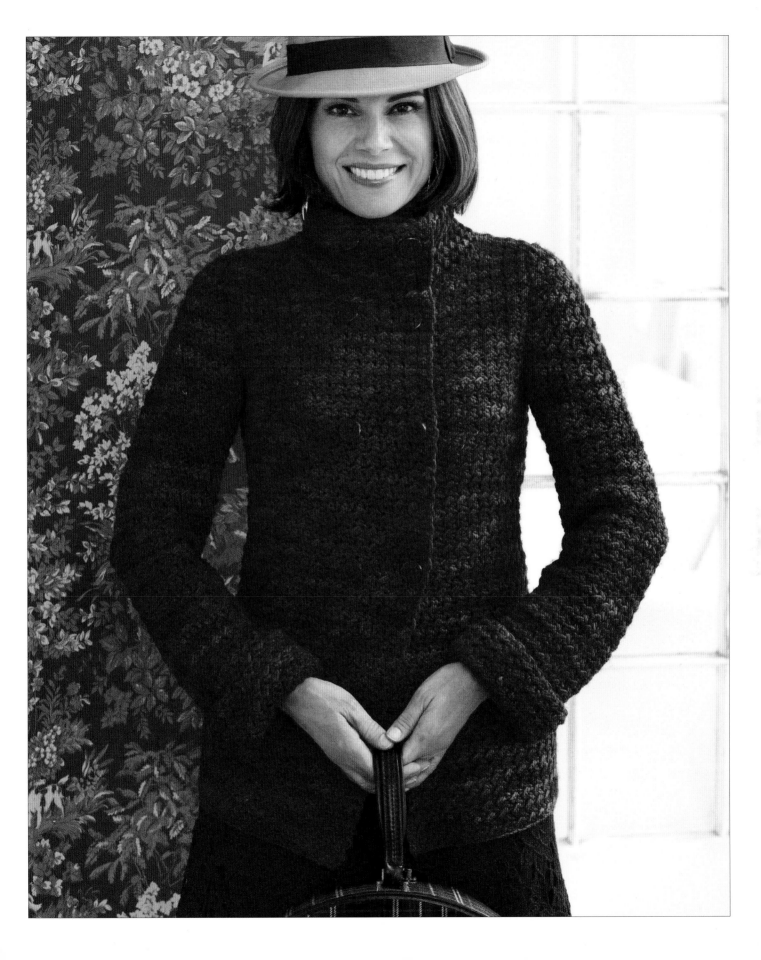

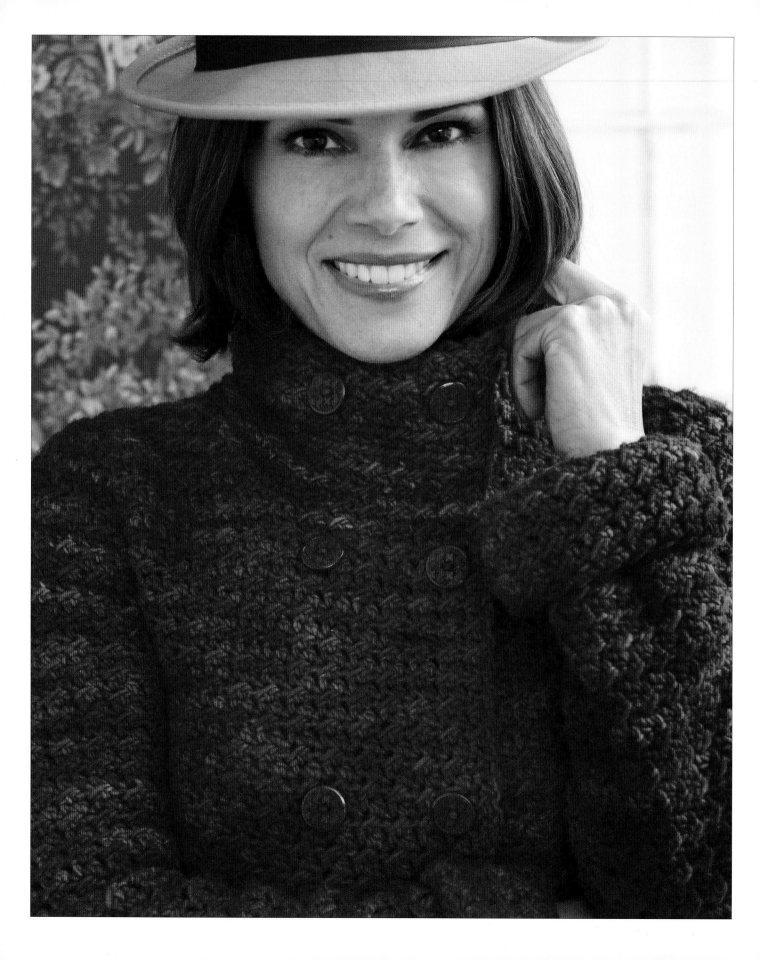

Work even in crinkle st until piece measures approx 23 (23½, 24, 24½, 25)"/58.5 (59.5, 61, 62, 63.5)cm from beg, end with a RS row. Fasten off.

NECK SHAPING

Next row (WS) Turn, sl st in first 15 (13, 15, 13, 15) sts, work in crinkle st as established to end—16 (18, 18, 22, 22) sts. **Note** First 14 (12, 14, 12, 14) sl sts of this row are not included in st count. Do not work into these sts when working next row.
Cont working in crinkle st as established AND dec 1 st at neck edge every row 6 times—10 (12, 12, 16, 16) sts.
Work even in crinkle st until piece measures same as back. Fasten off. Place markers for six buttons. Place first two markers ¾"/2cm down from beg of neck shaping and 2½"/6.5cm apart. Place next two markers 18 rows below first two. Place last two markers 18 rows below second set of two markers.

RIGHT FRONT

Note As you work the right front, each time the piece measures same length as left front to a button marker, make buttonhole at beg of next RS row as foll: Work in crinkle st over first 2 sts, ch 2, sk next 2 sts, work in crinkle st over next 7 sts, ch 2, sk next 2 sts, cont in crinkle st to end of row as instructed.
With smaller hook, ch 37 (39, 43, 45, 49).
Work crinkle st set-up row—36 (38, 42, 44, 48) sts.
Work even in crinkle st until piece measures approx 18½"/47cm from beg, end with a WS row.

ARMHOLE SHAPING

Next row (RS) Work in crinkle st as established to last 2 (4, 5, 6, 7) sts; leave last 2 (4, 5, 6, 7) sts unworked—34 (34, 37, 38, 41) sts.

Cont working in crinkle st as established AND dec 1 st at armhole edge every row 1 (1, 2, 0, 1) times. Then dec 1 st at armhole edge every other row 3 (3, 3, 4, 4) times—30 (30, 32, 34, 36) sts. Work even in crinkle st until piece measures approx 23 (23½, 24, 24½, 25)"/58.5 (59.5, 61, 62, 63.5)cm from beg, end with a RS row. Fasten off.

NECK SHAPING

Next Row (WS) Work in crinkle st as established to last 14 (12, 14, 12, 14) sts; leave last 14 (12, 14, 12, 14) sts unworked—16 (18, 18, 22, 22) sts.
Cont working in crinkle st as established AND dec 1 st at neck edge every row 6 times—10 (12, 12, 16, 16) sts.
Work even in crinkle st until piece measures same as back. Fasten off.

SLEEVE

With larger hook, ch 41 (41, 43, 47, 47).
Work crinkle st set-up row—40 (40, 42, 46, 46) sts.
Work even in crinkle st until piece measures approx 4"/10cm from beg, ending with a WS row. Change to smaller hook.
Work even in crinkle st until piece measures approx 22½"/57cm from beg, end with a WS row.

CAP SHAPING

Next row (RS) Turn, sl st in first 3 (5, 6, 7, 8) sts, work in crinkle st as established to last 2 (4, 5, 6, 7) sts; leave last 2 (4, 5, 6, 7) sts unworked—36 (32, 32, 34, 32) sts.
Cont working in crinkle st as established AND dec 1 st at beg and end of every 4th row 0 (3, 4, 3, 5) times. Then dec 1 st at beg and end of every other row 9 (4, 3, 5, 2) times—18 sts.
Next row Turn, sl st in first 3 sts, work in crinkle st as established to last 2 sts; leave last 2 sts unworked—14 sts.

Next row Turn, sl st in first 3 sts, work in crinkle st as established to last 2 sts; leave last 2 sts unworked—10 sts.
Fasten off.

FINISHING

Sew shoulder seams, leaving center 22 (20, 22, 20, 22) sts unsewn for back neck. Sew in sleeves. Sew side and sleeve seams. Fold lower 4"/10cm of sleeves back to form cuffs.

NECKBAND

With WS facing and smaller hook, join yarn with sl st in beg of left front neck edge, ch 2, work 86 sts in crinkle st evenly spaced around neck opening. Work even in crinkle st until neckband measures approx 3¼"/8cm from beg, end with a WS row.
Buttonhole row (RS) Work in crinkle st over first 2 sts, ch 2, sk next 2 sts, work in crinkle st over next 7 sts, ch 2, sk next 2 sts, work in crinkle st to end of row.
Work even in crinkle st until neckband measures approx 4"/10cm from beg. Fasten off. Sew buttons opposite buttonholes (where marked). ❤

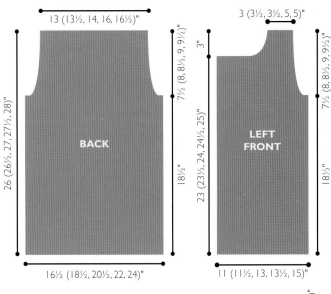

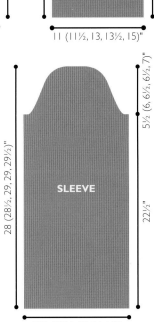

DEBBIE BLISS AND KATHY MERRICK

Scottie Pillow

Great Scot! This charming pillow cover features an argyle band between two rows of sweet Scottish terriers with ribbon and button accents.

■■□□

MEASUREMENTS
WIDTH
12"/30.5cm
HEIGHT
12"/30.5cm

MATERIALS
- 3 1¾oz/50g balls (each approx 115yd/105m) of Debbie Bliss/KFI *Rialto DK* (merino) in #12 scarlet (A) ③
- 1 ball each #03 black (B) and #09 apple (C)
- Size G/6 (4mm) crochet hook *or size to obtain gauge*
- Tapestry needle
- 12 buttons, ¼"/5mm diameter
- 2½yd/2.25m matching ribbon, ⅛"/2.5mm wide
- Sewing needle and thread in matching color
- 12"/30.5cm square pillow form

GAUGE
20 sts and 19 rnds to 4"/10cm over sc tbl using size G/6 (4mm) crochet hook.
➤ Take time to check gauge.

NOTES
1) Sc tbl is used throughout unless otherwise noted.
2) Pillow is worked in the round without turning and joining with sl st at the end of each round.
3) Each row of the chart is worked from right to left as you crochet.
4) When changing colors, work stitch until 2 loops remain on hook, then change to new color and draw through last 2 loops on hook.
5) Strand the color not used on wrong side of fabric, twisting strands every 4 or 5 stitches.

PILLOW
With A, ch 122, join with sl st in first ch to form a ring.
Rnd 1 (RS) Ch 1, sc in each ch around, sl st to first sc—122 sc.
Rnds 2–4 Ch 1, sc tbl in each sc around, sl st to first sc.
Rnds 5–17 Ch 1, *work 19-st rep of chart 1 in sc tbl 3 times, sc tbl in next 4 sc; rep from * once, sl st to first sc.
Rnds 18–21 Ch 1, sc tbl in each sc around with A, sl st to first sc.
Rnds 22–30 Ch 1, sc tbl in next 3 sc, work 9-st rep of chart 2 in

sc tbl, 13 times, sc tbl in last 2 sc with A, sl st to first sc.
Rnds 31–34 Ch 1, sc tbl in each sc around with A, sl st to first sc.
Rnds 35–47 Ch 1, *work 19-st rep of chart 1 in sc tbl, 3 times, sc tbl in next 4 sc; rep from * once, sl st to first sc.
Rnds 48–51 Ch 1, sc tbl in each sc around with A, sl st to first sc. Fasten off.

FINISHING
Block pillow to finished measurements. Using photo as guide, sew buttons to Scotties for eyes. Cut ribbon into 7"/18cm lengths. Loop ribbon around Scotties' collars, using a square knot to secure, and trim to desired length.

Turn pillow inside out with RS facing. Join A to top of pillow with sl st. Working through both sides of pillow at once, sl st in each st across (seaming top of pillow closed), fasten off. Turn pillow right side out. Insert pillow form. Using tapestry needle and A, whipstitch bottom of pillow closed. ❤

COLOR KEY
- ■ Scarlet (A)
- ▦ Black (B)
- ▨ Apple (C)

CHART 1

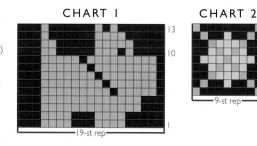

19-st rep

CHART 2

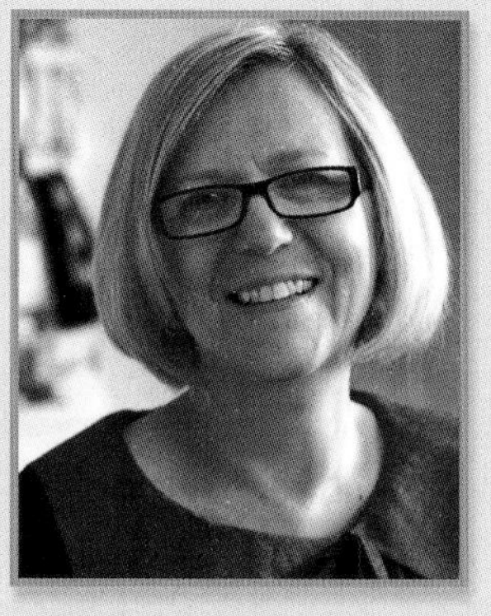

9-st rep

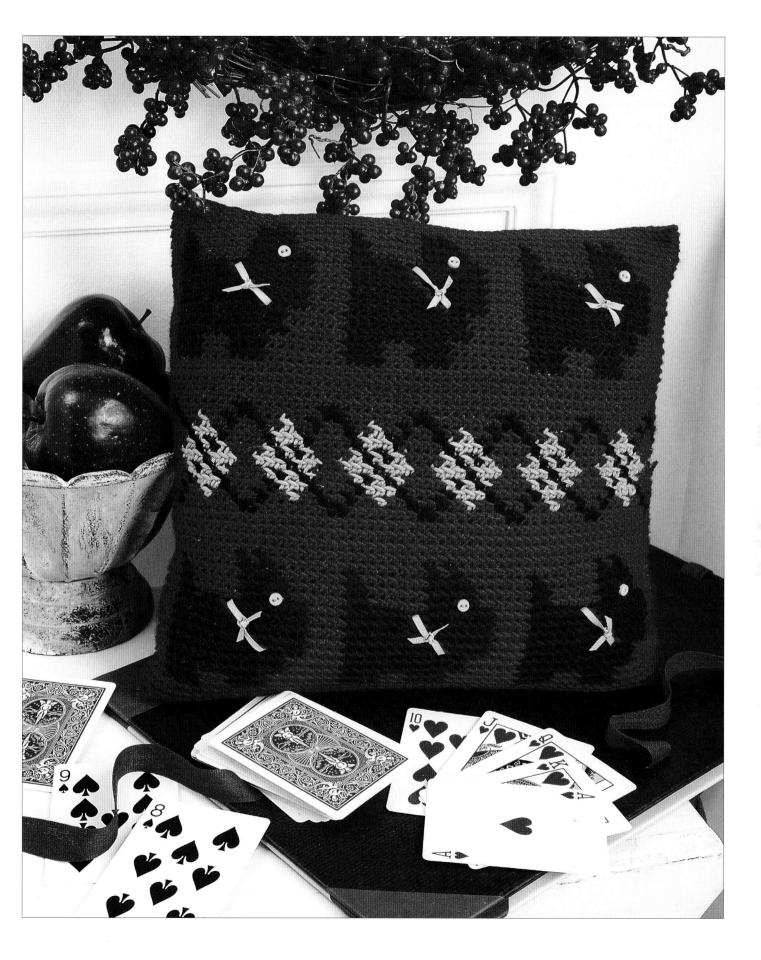

Flower Lace Scarf

An ethereal floral motif worked in a gorgeous beaded silk yarn feels luxurious on the neck, or around the shoulders as a capelet.

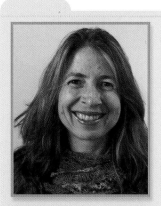

■■■□

SIZE
Instructions are written for one size.

MEASUREMENTS
LENGTH 44"/112cm
WIDTH 7½"/19cm

MATERIALS
• 1 1¾oz/50g hank (each approx 160yd/146m) of Artyarns *Beaded Silk Light* (silk/glass beads) in #244G red with gold beads (3)
• Size H/8 (5mm) crochet hook *or size to obtain gauge*
• Tapestry needle

GAUGE
Entire width of row 6 = 7½"/19cm; rows 1–9 = 6"/15cm long over pattern using size H/8 (5mm) crochet hook.
➤ Take time to check gauge.

SCARF
Ch 22.
Row 1 (RS) 7 tr in 4th ch from hook, sk 3 ch, sc in next ch, ch 9, sk 7 ch, sc in next ch, ch 5, sk 3 ch, dc in next 3 ch—1 tr group.
Row 2 Ch 3 (counts as dc throughout), turn, dc in next 2 dc, ch 5, sc in next sc, ch 5, sc in ch-9 sp, ch 5, sc in next sc, ch 5, sk 3 tr, sc in next tr, ch 5, sc in last tr—5 ch-5 sps.
Row 3 Ch 5, turn, 7 tr in first sc, sk next ch-5 sp, sc in next sc, sk next ch-5 sp, 7 tr in next sc, sk next ch-5 sp, sc in next sc, ch 9, sk next sc, dc in next 2 dc, dc in top of t-ch— 2 tr groups.
Row 4 Ch 3, turn, dc in next 2 dc, ch 5, sc in ch-9 sp, ch 5, sc in next sc, ch 5, sk 3 tr, sc in next tr, ch 5, sk 3 tr, sc in next sc, ch 5, sk 3 tr, sc in next tr, ch 5, sc in top of t-ch—6 ch-5 sps.
Row 5 Ch 5, turn, 7 tr in first sc, sk next ch-5 sp, sc in next sc, ch 9, sk next sc, sc in next sc, sk next ch-5 sp, 7 tr in next sc, sk next ch-5 sp, sc in next sc, ch 5, dc in next 2 dc, dc in top of t-ch.
Row 6 Ch 3, turn, dc in next 2 dc, ch 5, sk ch-5 sp, sc in next sc, ch 5, sk 3 tr, sc in next tr, ch 5, sc in next sc, ch 5, sc in ch-9 sp, ch 5, sc in next sc, ch 5, sk 3 tr, sc in next tr.

Row 7 Turn, sk first sc, sk next ch-5 sp, 7 tr in next sc, sk next ch-5 sp, sc in next sc, sk next ch-5 sp, 7 tr in next sc, sk next ch-5 sp, ch 9, sk next sc, dc in next 2 dc, dc in top of t-ch.
Row 8 Ch 3, turn, dc in next 2 dc, ch 5, sc in ch-9 sp, ch 5, sc in next sc, ch 5, sk 3 tr, sc in next tr, ch 5, sc in next sc, ch 5, sk 3 tr, sc in next tr— 5 ch-5 sps.
Row 9 Turn, sk first sc, sk next ch-5 sp, 7 tr in next sc, sk next ch-5 sp, sc in next sc, ch 9, sk next sc, sc in next sc, ch 5, dc in next 2 dc, dc in top of t-ch—1 tr group.
Rep rows 2–9 seven times more, do not fasten off.

FINISHING
Turn work 90 degrees to start working on edge of scarf.
Row 1 Ch 2, sk 2 rows, *sc around post of next row end, ch 5, sk next row end; rep from * to last row end, sc around post of last row end, ch 5, sc in foundation ch—32 ch-5 sps.
Row 2 Ch 8, turn, sk first sc, *sc in next sc, ch 8, sk next ch-5 sp; rep from * across, sc in last sc, fasten off.
Block lightly to measurements, pinning out points of motifs.♥

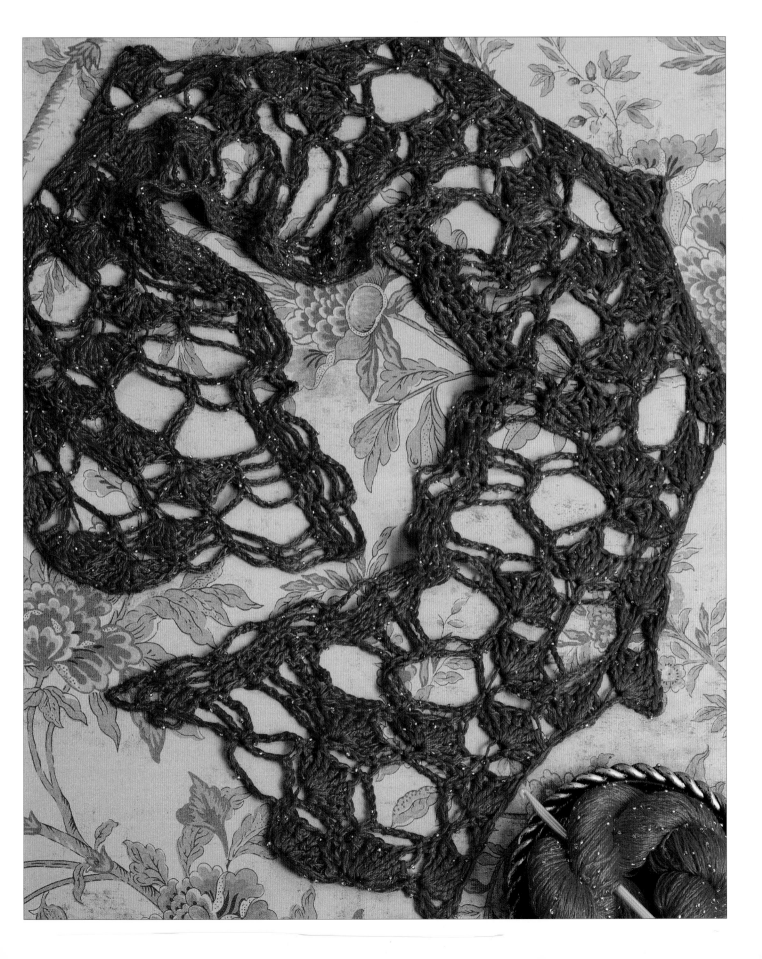

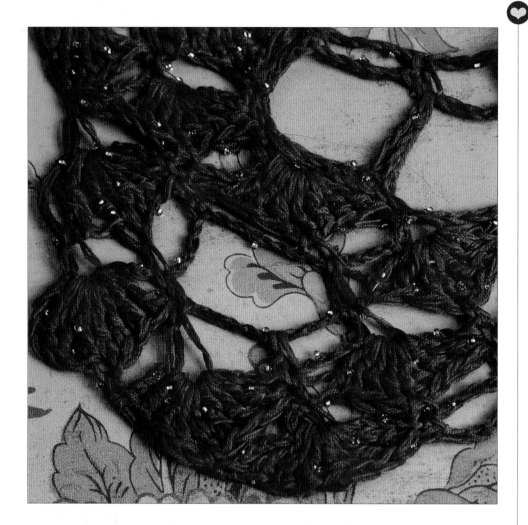

STITCH KEY

o	ch
+	sc
T	dc
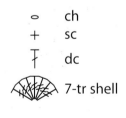	7-tr shell

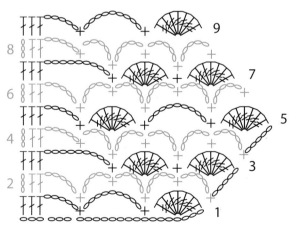

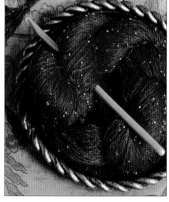

IRIS'S TIP
KEEP EXERCISE FROM
BECOMING A BORE
by rotating among lifting
weights, practicing yoga,
and doing cardio.

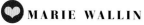

MARIE WALLIN

Eyelet-Stripe Tunic

This oversized tunic-length sweater crocheted in an ultra-soft wool and mohair blend features stripes of alternating stitch patterns that flow seamlessly into the sleeves.

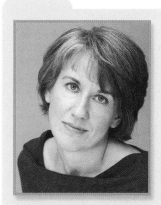

◀■■■▭

SIZES
Instructions are written for size X-Small. Changes for Small, Medium, Large, and X-Large are in parentheses. (Shown in size Small.)

MEASUREMENTS
BUST
45 (47, 51, 56, 61)"/114 (119.5, 129.5, 142, 156)cm
LENGTH
25 (26, 27, 27½, 28½)"/63.5 (66, 68.5, 70, 72.5)cm

MATERIALS
• 9 (10, 10, 11, 12) 1¾oz/50g balls (each approx 153yd/140m) of Rowan *Kid Classic* (lambswool/kid mohair/polyamide) in #847 cherry red (**4**)
• Size H/8 (5mm) crochet hook *or size to obtain gauge*
• Tapestry needle

GAUGE
21 sts = 4"/10cm and 2 pat reps (30 rows) = 13¼"/33.5cm over pat using size H/8 (5mm) crochet hook.
➤ Take time to check gauge.

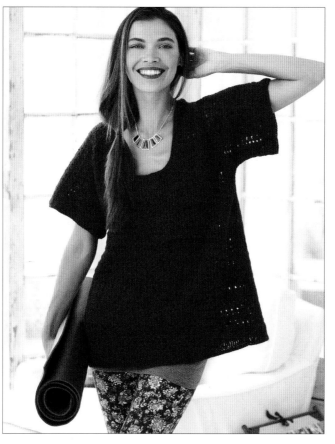

STITCH GLOSSARY
Cl (cluster) [Yo, insert hook in indicated st, draw up a lp, yo, draw through 2 lps] 3 times, yo, draw through all 4 lps on hook.
V-st (V-stitch) [dc, ch 1, dc] in indicated st.
trtr2tog (triple treble 2 together) *Yo 4 times, insert hook, draw up lp, [yo and pull through 2 lps] 4 times; rep from *, yo and draw through all 3 lps on hook.
trtr3tog (triple treble 3 together)

*Yo 4 times, insert hook, draw up lp, [yo and pull through 2 lps] 4 times, rep from * twice, yo and draw through all 4 lps on hook.

BACK
Row 1 (WS) Ch 114 (126, 138, 150, 165), sc in 2nd ch from hook, sc in each ch across, turn—113 (125, 137, 149, 164) sc.
Row 2 Ch 6 (counts as trtr, here and throughout), trtr in each sc across, turn.

Row 3 Ch 3 (counts as 1 dc here and throughout), [sk 2 trtr, V-st in next trtr] across to last trtr, sk trtr, dc in top of t-ch, turn—112 (124, 136, 148, 163) sts.

Row 4 Ch 4 (counts as dc, ch 1 here and throughout), [cl in next ch-sp, ch 2] across to last ch-sp, cl in ch-sp, ch 1, dc in top of t-ch, turn—113 (125, 137, 149, 164) sts.

Row 5 Ch 3, V-st in each cl across, dc in 3rd st of t-ch, turn.

Rows 6–10 Rep rows 4 and 5 twice, then row 4 once.

Row 11 Ch 6, trtr in ch-sp, [trtr in cl, 2 trtr in next ch sp] across to last ch-sp, trtr in ch-sp, trtr in 3rd st of t-ch, turn.

Row 12 Ch 1, sc in each st across, turn.

Row 13 Ch 4, [sk 1 sc, dc in next sc, ch 1] across to last 2 sc, dc in last 2 sc, turn.

Row 14 Ch 4, [cl in next ch-sp, ch 2, sk 2 sts, cl in next dc, 2 ch, sk 2 sts] across, ending with ch 1, dc in 3rd st of t-ch, turn.

Row 15 Ch 1, sc in dc, sc in ch-sp, [sc in cl, 2 sc in next ch-sp] across, ending with 1 sc in last ch-sp, sc in 3rd st of t-ch, turn.

Row 16 Ch 1, sc in each sc across, turn.

Rep rows 2–16 for pat.

Rows 17–39 (40, 40, 41, 42) Work in pat for 23 (24, 24, 25, 26) rows, ending after a pat row 9 [10, 10, 11, 12].

SLEEVE SHAPING
Join a new piece of yarn in the 1st st of the last row, ch 18, fasten off.

Size X-Small only
Row 40 Ch 21, cl in 6th ch from hook (counts as ch 1, dc, ch 1), [ch 2, sk 2 ch, cl in next ch] 5 times, [ch 2, cl in next ch-sp] across to last ch-sp, ch 2, sk next 2 sts [cl in next ch, 2 ch, sk 2 ch] 5 times, cl in next ch, ch 1, sk 1 ch, dc in last ch, turn—149 sts.**

Sizes Small and Medium only
Row 41 Ch 23, trtr in 7th ch from hook, trtr in next 16 ch and each st across, turn—161 (173) sts.**

Size Large only
Row 42 Ch 19, sc in 2nd ch from hook, sc in each st across, turn—185 sts.**

Size X-Large only
Row 43 Ch 22, dc in 6th ch from hook (counts as ch 1, dc, ch 1), [ch 1, sk 1 st, dc in next st] across to last 2 ch, dc in last 2 ch, turn—200 sts.**

All sizes
Cont in pat as established for 15 [15, 17, 19, 19] rows, ending after a pat row 10 [11, 13, 16, 2].

SHAPE NECK
Size X-Small only
Row 56 Work 49 sts of pat row 11, dtr in same ch-sp as last trtr, tr in next cl, (dc, hdc) in next ch-sp, sc in next cl, sl st in next ch-sp, fasten off. Sk next 12 ch-sps, join yarn in next ch-sp, sc in next cl, (hdc, dc) in next ch-sp, tr in next cl, (dtr, trtr) in next ch-sp, cont in pat row 11 across, fasten off.

Size Small only
Row 57a Ch 1, sc in next 56 trtr, sc2tog, turn, leaving rem sts unworked—57 sc.

Row 58a Ch 4, sk sc2tog and next sc, dc in next sc, [ch 1, sk 1 sc, dc in next sc] across, turn—56 sts.

Row 59a Ch 4, [sk next 2 sts, cl in next dc, ch 2, sk 2 sts, cl in next ch-sp, ch 2] 9 times, omitting last ch 2, ch 1, dc in t-ch, fasten off. Return to row 57, sk center 55 trtr, join yarn in next trtr.

Row 57b Ch 1, sc2tog in same st as join and next trtr, sc in next 56 sts, turn—57 sc.

Row 58b Ch 4, sk 2 sc, dc in next sc, [ch 1, sk 1 sc, dc in next sc] 26 times, sk 1 sc, dc in next st, turn—56 sts.

Row 59b Ch 4, [sk 2 sts, cl in next dc, ch 2, sk 2 sts, cl in next ch-sp, ch 2] 9 times, omitting last ch 2, ch 1, dc in t-ch, fasten off.

Size Medium only
Row 58a Ch 4, sk 2 dc, [cl in next ch-sp, ch 2, sk 2 sts, cl in next dc, ch 2, sk 2 sts] 10 times, omitting last ch, sk 1 ch, dc2tog skipping ch-sp, turn, leaving rem sts unworked—62 sts.

Row 59a Ch 1, sc2tog, [sc in next cl, 2 sc in next ch-sp] 19 times, sc in next cl, sc in next ch-sp, dc in 3rd st of t-ch, turn—61 sts.

Row 60a Ch 1, sc in next 59 sc, sc2tog, turn—60 sc.

Row 61a Ch 1, sc in each st across, fasten off.
Return to row 58, sk center 22 dc, join yarn in next dc.

Row 58b Ch 3, dc in next ch-sp, ch 1, [cl in next ch-sp, ch 2, sk 2 sts, cl in next dc, ch 2, sk 2 sts] 10 times, omitting last ch, dc in 3rd st of t-ch, turn—62 sts.

Row 59b Ch 1, sc in dc, sc in ch-sp, [sc in next cl, 2 sc in next ch-sp] 19 times, sc in next cl, sk ch, sc2tog, turn—61 sts.

Row 60b Ch 1, sc2tog, sc in next 59 sc, turn—60 sts.

Row 61b Ch 1, sc in each st across, fasten off.

Size Large only
Row 62 Ch 6, trtr in next 65 sc, dtr in next sc, tr in next sc, dc in next sc, hdc in next sc, sc in next sc, sl st in next sc, fasten off. Sk 53 sc, join yarn in next sc, sc in next sc, hdc in next sc, dc in next sc, tr in next sc, dtr in next sc, trtr in next sc, trtr in each st across, fasten off.

Size X-Large only
Row 63a Ch 3, sk 2 trtr, [V-st in next trtr, sk 2 trtr] 23 times, dc in next trtr turn, leaving rem sts unworked.

Row 64a Ch 3, [cl in next ch-sp, 2 ch] 23 times, cl in next ch-sp, ch 1, dc in 3rd st of t-ch, fasten off—73 sts.

Return to row 63, sk center 50 trtr, join yarn in next trtr.

Row 63b Ch 3, sk trtr, [V-st in next trtr, sk 2 trtr] 23 times, V-st in next trtr, sk 1 trtr, dc in t-ch, turn.

Row 64b Ch 4, [cl in next ch sp, ch 2] 23 times, cl in next ch-sp, dc in t-ch, fasten off—73 sts.

FRONT
Work as for back to **.
Work 1 (3, 5, 5, 6) rows, ending after pat row 11 (14, 16, 2, 4).

SHAPE NECK
Size X-small only
Row 42a Ch 1, sc in 1st 60 trtr, sc2tog, turn, leaving rem sts unworked—61 sts.

Row 43a Ch 3, sk 3 sts, dc in next sc, [ch 1, sk 1 sc, dc in next sc] across to last 2 sc, dc in last 2 sc, turn—60 sts.

Row 44a Ch 4, [cl in next dc, ch 2, sk 2 sts, cl in next ch-sp, ch 2, sk 2 sts] 9 times, dc2tog skipping ch-sp, turn—57 sts.

Row 45a Ch 1, sc2tog, sc in same ch-sp, [sc in cl, 2 sc in next ch-sp] across ending with 1 sc in last ch-sp, sc in 3rd st of t-ch, turn—56 sts.
Work rows 46b–56b below, fasten off.
Return to row 42, sk center 25 trtr, join yarn in next trtr.

Row 42b Ch 1, sc2tog in trtr where yarn was joined and next trtr, sc in each st across, turn—61 sts.

Row 43b Rep pat row 13, ending with dc2tog in last 2 sts, turn–60 sts.

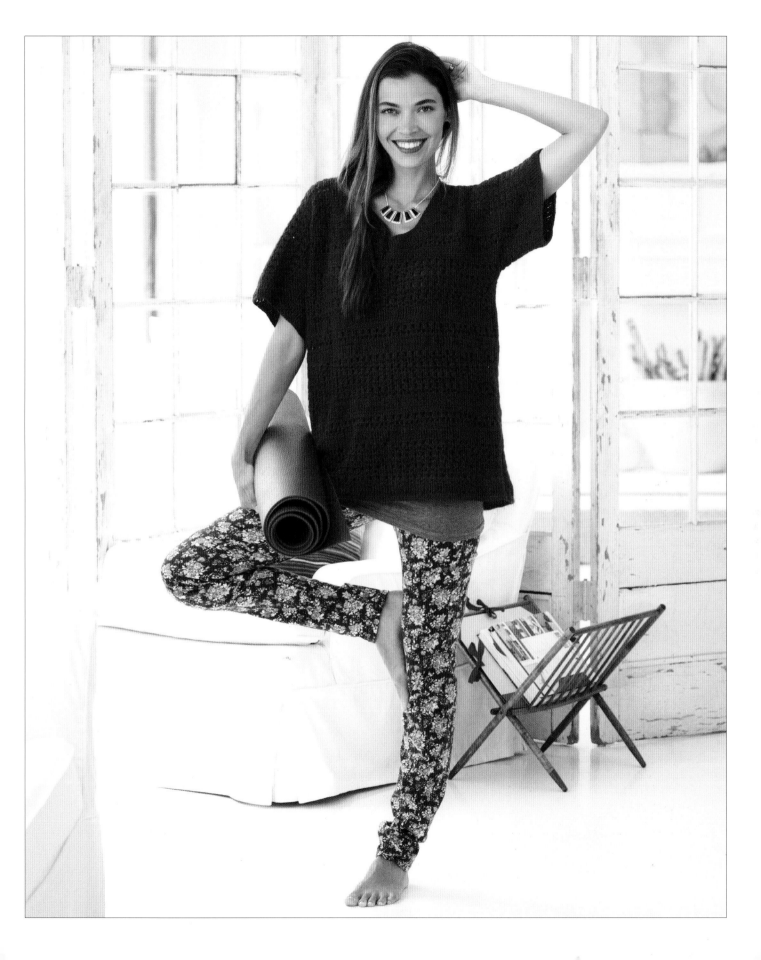

Row 44b Ch 3, dc in next dc, ch 2, sk 2 sts, [cl in next ch-sp, ch 2, sk 2 sts, cl in next dc, 2 ch, sk 2 sts] across, ending with ch 1, dc in 3rd st of t-ch, turn.

Row 45b Rep pat row 15 to last cl, sc in next ch-sp, sc2tog in same ch-sp and next dc, turn—56 sts. Work rows 46a–56a below, fasten off.

Size Small only

Row 45a Ch 1, sc in dc, sc in ch-sp, [sc in cl, 2 sc in next ch-sp] 21 times, sc in cl, sc in ch-sp, sc2tog in ch-sp and next cl, turn, leaving rem sts unworked—68 sts.

Row 46a Ch 1, sc2tog, sc in each st across, turn.

Row 47a Rep pat row 2 to last 3 sts, trtr3tog, turn. Work rows 48a–59a below, fasten off.

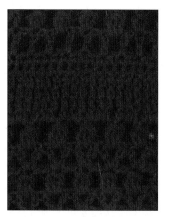

Return to row 45, sk cl used for last st of 1st side of neck and next 7 cl, join yarn in next cl and cont as foll:

Row 45b Ch 1, sc2tog over cl where yarn was rejoined and next ch-sp, sc in same ch-sp, [sc in cl, 2 sc in next ch-sp] across ending with 1 sc in last ch-sp, sc in 3rd st of t-ch, turn.

Row 46b Ch 1, sc in first 54 sc, sc2tog, turn—55 sts.

Row 47b Ch 6, sk sc2tog, trtr2tog, trtr in each st across, turn—54 sts. Work rows 48b–59b below, fasten off.

Size Medium only

Row 47a Ch 6, trtr in 1st 70 sc, trtr3tog, turn, leaving rem sts unworked—71 sts.

Row 48a Ch 3 (does *not* count as st), sk trtr3tog and next trtr, V-st in next trtr, [sk 2 trtr, V-st in next trtr] across, dc in 3rd st of t-ch, turn.

Work rows 49a–61a below, fasten off.

Return to row 47, sk center 27 sc, join yarn in next sc and cont as foll:

Row 47b Ch 6, trtr2tog, trtr in each st across, turn—71 sts.

Row 48b Ch 3, [sk 2 trtr, V-st in next trtr] 16 times, sk 2 trtr, dc in next trtr, ch 1, dc2tog in same trtr as last dc and trtr2tog, turn. Work rows 49b–61b below, fasten off.

Size Large only

Row 48a Ch 3, [sk 2 trtr, V-st in next trtr] 25 times, sk 2 trtr, dc in next 2 trtr, turn, leaving rem sts unworked.

Row 49a Rep pat row 4, skipping last V-st.

Row 50a Rep pat row 4. Work rows 51a–62a below, fasten off.

Return to row 48, sk center 27 trtr, join yarn in next trtr and cont as foll:

Row 48b Ch 3, cont as for pat row 3.

Row 49b Rep pat row 4, ending by skipping last ch-sp, dc in dc2tog, turn.

Row 50b–62b Rep rows 50a–62a. Fasten off.

Size X-Large only

Row 50a Ch 3, V-st in next 28 cl, dc in next cl, turn, leaving rem sts unworked.

Row 51a Rep pat row 4.

Row 52a, 54a Ch 3, dc in 1st cl, V-st in each cl across, dc in 3rd st of t-ch, turn.

Row 53a, 55a Rep pat row 4 across, turn.

Row 56a Rep pat row 11, fasten off for size X-Small.

Row 57a Ch 1, sc in each st across, turn.

Row 58a and 59a Rep pat rows 13 and 14. Fasten off for size Small.

Rows 60a and 61a Rep pat rows 15 and 16. Fasten off for size Medium.

Row 62a Ch 6, trtr in each sc across. Fasten off for size Large.

Row 63a Ch 3, [sk 2 trtr, V-st in next trtr] 23 times, sk 2 trtr, dc in next trtr, ch 1, dc in next trtr, turn.

Row 64a Ch 3, [cl in next V-st, ch 2] across, dc in top of t-ch, fasten off for size X-Large.

Return to row 50, sk center 9 ch-sps, join yarn in next cl and cont as foll:

Row 50b Rep pat row 5.

Row 51b Ch 4, [cl in next ch-sp, ch 2] 28 times, dc in top of t-ch, turn.

Row 52b Ch 3, dc in 1st cl, V-st in each cl across, dc in top of t-ch, across, turn.

Row 53b Ch 4, [cl in next ch-sp, ch 2] 27 times, ch 1, dc in top of t-ch, turn.

Row 54b Rep pat row 5.

Row 55b Ch 4 [cl in next ch-sp, ch 2] 26 times, ch 2, sk V-st, dc in next dc, turn.

Row 56b Ch 6, trtr2tog in next ch-sp, [trtr in next cl, 2 trtr in next ch-sp] 25 times, trtr in next cl, ch-sp, and 3rd st t-ch, turn.

Row 57b Ch 1, sc in 1st 77 trtr, sc2tog, turn—78 sts.

Row 58b Ch 4, sk 3 sc, dc in next sc, (ch 1, sk 1 sc, dc in next sc) 37 times, turn—77 sts.

Row 59b Ch 4, [cl in next ch-sp, ch 2, sk 2 sts, cl in next dc, ch 2, sk 2 sts] 12 times, cl in next ch -sp, dc in 3rd st of t-ch, turn.

Row 60b Ch 1, sc2tog over dc and cl, (2 sc in next ch-sp, sc in next bo) 24 times, sc in next ch-sp, sc in 3rd st of t-ch, turn.

Row 61b Ch 1, sc in 1st 73 sc, sc2tog, turn—74 sts.

Row 62b Ch 6, trtr in each dc across, turn—73 sts.

Row 63b Ch 3, [sk 2 trtr, V-st in next trtr] 23 times, sk 2 trtr, dc in next trtr, ch 1, dc in last trtr, turn.

Row 64b Rep pat row 4, fasten off for size X-Large.

FINISHING

Block lightly to measurements. Sew shoulder seams.

NECKBAND

Rnd 1 (RS) Join yarn at seam, ch 1, sc evenly around neck opening, sl st in 1st sc to join.

Rnd 2 Ch 6, trtr in each sc around, working trtr2tog as required to ensure neckband lies flat, end with sl st in top of t-ch at beg of round.

Rnd 3 Ch 1, sc in each st around, sl st in 1st sc to join, fasten off. Sew side and sleeve seams. Work each cuff as for neckband.❤

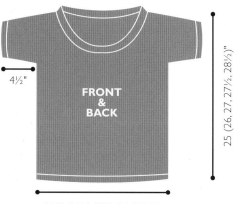

4½"

FRONT & BACK

25 (26, 27, 27½, 28½)"

21½ (23½, 25½, 28, 30½)"

❤ NORA J. BELLOWS WITH JANET BRANI

Beaded Felted Bag

Made with a bag kit and sturdy felted wool, this purse is both useful and enchanting, with beading, a padlock charm, and a long bottom tassel.

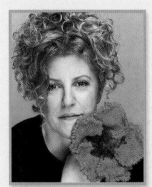

MEASUREMENTS
WIDTH (AFTER FELTING)
4½"/11.5cm
HEIGHT (AFTER FELTING)
6½"/16.5cm

MATERIALS
• 1 4oz/113g hank (each approx 250yd/229m) of Stonehedge Fiber Mill *Shepherd's Wool Worsted* (wool) in Christmas red or hot pink (4)
• Size H/8 (5mm) crochet hook *or size to obtain gauge*
• Sharp sewing needle
• Stitch markers
• Noni *Heart on My Sleeve* bag kit: Includes tiny frame, 10" (25cm) chain, tiny heart locket and key, color-matched seed beads, nylon beading thread, and decorative tassel
• Tapestry needle or metal double-pointed needle
• Beading needle
• Clear-drying fabric glue

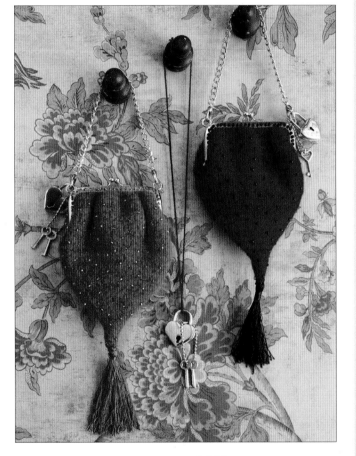

GAUGE
14 sc and 12 rows = 4"/10 worked tfl only, before felting, using size H/8 (5mm) crochet hook.
➤ Take time to check gauge.

STITCH GLOSSARY
Sc2tog (single crochet 2 together) Pull up a lp in each of 2 indicated sts, yo and draw through all 3 lps on hook.

NOTES
1) Bag is worked from the top down. Flaps are started separately, then joined together.
2) After flaps are joined, bag is worked in rnds, turning work after each rnd.
3) Beg with rnd 19, bag is worked in spiral fashion, with no joining or turning.

NORA'S STORY
Nora Bellows had no idea a job in her local yarn shop would become a career. But customers began clamoring for her innovative felted bags—and no wonder! As Nora says, they're not just useful; they're a fashion statement. Nora started teaching people to make the bags and selling patterns under her Noni label. These days, she travels around teaching and helping crafters add their own one-of-a-kind touch. Nora has had friends affected by heart disease and was glad to contribute to *Crochet Red*. She keeps her family healthy by tending a garden, which is excellent exercise and ensures that home-grown vegetables play a starring role in her cooking.

JANET'S STORY
Georgia native Janet Brani, who translated Nora's pattern into crochet, learned to crochet when she was just eight. Luckily, neither Janet nor her loved ones have been affected by heart disease, and she keeps healthy by walking her dog and making heart-healthy soups full of veggies and whole grains.

BAG

FIRST FLAP
Ch 15.

Row 1 (RS) Sc in 2nd ch from hook and in each ch to end—14 sc. Place marker (pm) for RS.

Row 2 Ch 1, sc tfl in each st to end.

Row 3 Ch 1, (sc tfl, sc tbl, sc tfl) in each sc to end—42 sc.

Row 4 Ch 1, sc tfl in each st to end.

Row 5 Ch 1, sc tfl in each st to end, pm in last st. Fasten off.

SECOND FLAP
Work same as first flap through row 4.

Row 5 Ch 1, sc tfl in each st to end.

Row 6 Ch 1, [sc tfl in each of next 4 sts, sc2tog tfl over next 2 sts] 7 times, pm in first st of row, do *not* turn—35 sc. Join to first flap as foll: with WS facing, sc into marked st (last st of row 5), sc tfl in each of next 3 sts, sc2tog tfl over next 2 sts, [sc tfl in each of next 4 sts, sc2tog tfl over next 2 sts] 6 times, do *not* turn—35 sc on first flap, 70 sc total. Being careful not to twist pieces, join to second flap with sl st in marked st (first st of row 6), turn. Beg working in rnds, turning after each rnd, as foll:

Rnd 7 Ch 1, sc in each st around, sl st in first sc, turn—70 sts.

Rnd 8 Ch 1, [sc in each of next 3 sc, sc2tog over next 2 sts] 14 times, sl st in first sc, turn—56 sts.

Rnd 9 Ch 1, sc around, sl st in first sc, turn.

Rnd 10 Ch 1, [sc in each of next 5 sc, sc2tog over next 2 sts] 8 times, sl st in first sc, turn—48 sts.

Rnd 11 Ch 1, sc around, sl st in first sc, turn.

Rnd 12 Ch 1, [sc in each of next 4 sc, sc2tog over next 2 sts] 8 times, sl st in first sc, turn—40 sts.

Rnd 13 Ch 1, sc around, sl st in first sc, turn.

Rnd 14 Ch 1, [sc in each of the next 3 sc, sc2tog over next 2 sts] 8 times, sl st in first sc, turn—32 sts.

Rnd 15 Ch 1, sc around, sl st in first sc, turn.

Rnd 16 Ch 1, [sc in each of the next 2 sc, sc2tog over next 2 sts] 8 times, sl st in first sc, turn—24 sts.

Rnd 17 Ch 1, sc around, sl st in first sc, turn.

Rnd 18 Ch 1, [sc in each of the next 2 sc, sc2tog over next 2 sts] 6 times, sl st in first sc, turn—18 sts.

Work the following rnd in a continuous spiral without joining or turning:

Next rnd Ch 1, [sc in each of the next 2 sc, sc2tog] 4 times, sc in each of the next 2 sc, sc2tog tbl over next 2 sc, [sc tbl in each of the next 2 sc, sc2tog tbl over next 2 sc] 9 times, pull up a lp tbl in each of 3 rem sts, yo and draw through all lps on hook, ch 1. Fasten off.

FINISHING

MACHINE FELTING
1) Use a low water setting and hottest temperature in a top-loading washing machine. Add small amount of laundry detergent and jeans or towels for agitation.

2) Place bag in a lingerie bag or zippered pillowcase and add to machine. Check the felting progress frequently, removing bag when the individual stitches are no longer visible and bag is felted to the desired size.

3) Place in cool water to stop the felting process and remove suds. Remove from lingerie bag and roll gently in towel to remove excess water.

4) Block and shape while wet. Pin into shape or stuff with plastic bags, and allow to air dry completely.

GLUE BAG INTO FRAME
Apply clear-drying fabric glue (instant-bond glues are not recommended) into the "slot" of purse frame. Press flap edges into the slot with a tapestry needle. Keep flaps in place while the glue dries with long (snug) basting stitches that go through the purse fabric and around frame. Remove basting stitches once glue has dried.

SEW BAG INTO FRAME
Use a needle and beading thread to sew flaps to the purse frame as foll: beg on inside of purse, *bring threaded needle through felt, through a metal purse frame hole, and through a bead. To reach the next sew-hole, angle the needle toward that hole as you put it back through the same frame hole the needle just came out of. Pull snug. Your needle is now on the inside of the bag. You can also put a bead on the thread here on the inside. Again, angle the needle toward the next sew-hole as you place the needle through the bag almost where it came out. Rep from * until each hole on frame exterior is filled with a bead. Finish off thread with a knot and cut.

APPLY BEADS AND TASSEL
Use a double strand of beading thread and a beading needle to apply seed beads one at a time to the surface of the bag in the arrangement of your choice. Place a tassel on the tail using the tassel loop. ❤

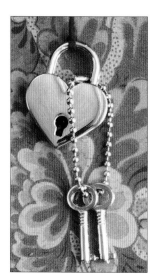

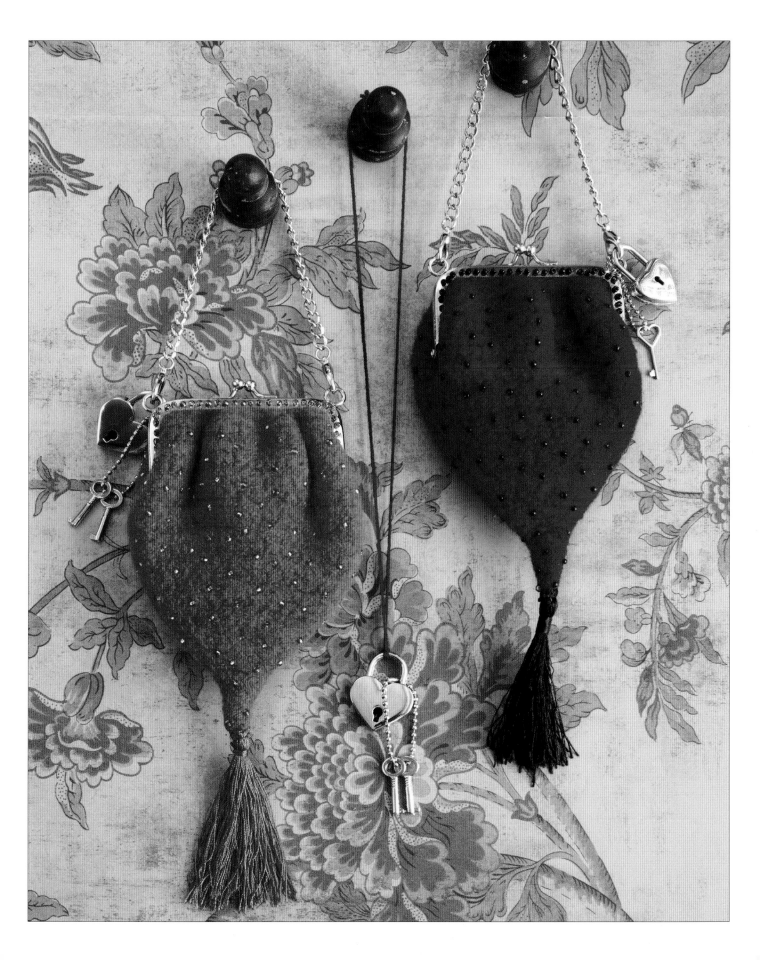

Heart-Shaped Coat

This showstopping sweater is all ▌ drama and all heart, with deep textures, asymmetrical fronts and back, and a velvet ribbon woven through the collar.

■■■■■

SIZES
Instructions are written for size Small. Changes for Medium, Large, and X-Large are in parentheses. (Shown in size Small.)

MEASUREMENTS
BUST 34 (38½, 42¾, 47⅛)"/86.5 (97.5, 108.5, 119.5)cm
BOTTOM EDGE 61¼ (65¾, 70, 74½)"/155.5 (167, 177.5, 189)cm
BACK LENGTH (NOT INCLUDING COLLAR) 15 (15, 17, 17)"/38 (38, 43, 43)cm

MATERIALS
• 10 (11, 12, 13) 3½oz/100g hanks (each approx 220yd/201m) of Cascade Yarns *220 Superwash* (superwash wool) in #893 ruby (4)
• One each sizes H/8 and I/9 (5 and 5.5mm) crochet hook *or size to obtain gauge*
• Stitch marker
• Tapestry needle
• 2 yards of ⅜" velvet ribbon
• 3 buttons, 1⅛" diameter (shown: JHB Buttons by Nicky Epstein, #93366 Lancelot)

GAUGES
2 scales and 8 rows = 4"/10cm by 3¾"/9.5cm over crocodile st using size I/9 (5.5mm) crochet hook.

16 sts and 10 rows = 4"/10cm in FPdc using size H/8 (5mm) crochet hook.
➤Take time to check gauges.

STITCH GLOSSARY
FPdc (front post double crochet)
Yo, insert hook from front to back to front around post of indicated st, draw up a lp, [yo and draw through 2 lps on hook] twice.
BPdc (back post double crochet)
Yo, insert hook from back to front to back around post of indicated st, draw up a lp, [yo and draw through 2 lps on hook] twice.
FPtr (front post treble crochet)
Yo twice, insert hook from front to back to front around post of indicated st, draw up a lp, [yo and draw through 2 lps on hook] 3 times.
BPtr (back post treble crochet)
Yo twice, insert hook from back to front to back around post of indicated st, draw up a lp, [yo and draw through 2 lps on hook] 3 times.

CROCODILE STITCH
Ch a multiple of 6 plus 4.
Row 1 (RS) 2 tr in 4th ch from hook, *ch 2, sk 2 ch, 2 tr in next ch; rep from * to end.
Row 2 Ch 3, turn (turn work 90 degrees to crochet around prev tr on row below), *5 tr around post of first tr of 2-tr group from top to base, ch 1, 5 tr around post of second tr of 2-tr group from base to top (scale made), sk next 2-tr group; rep from * to last 2-tr group, 5 tr around

post of first tr of 2-tr group from top to base, ch 1, 5 tr around post of second tr of 2-tr group from base to top.
Row 3 Ch 3, turn, *2 tr bet next 2-tr group (in center of scale), ch 2, 2 tr bet next 2-tr group (crochet between tr of unworked 2-tr group below and ALSO catch the ch-2 between scales), ch 2; rep from * to last 2-tr group, 2 tr bet next 2-tr group.
Row 4 Ch 3, turn (turn work 90 degrees to crochet around prev tr on row below), *sk next 2-tr group, 5 tr around post of first tr of 2-tr group from top to base, ch 1, 5 tr around post of second tr of 2-tr group from base to top; rep from * to last 2-tr group, sk last 2-tr group.
Row 5 Ch 3, turn, 2 tr bet first skipped 2-tr group below and ALSO crochet around last tr of prev scale, *ch 2, 2 tr bet next 2-tr group (in center of scale), ch 2, 2 tr bet next 2-tr group (crochet between last tr of next scale and first tr of prev scale, catching ch-2 bet scales); rep from * to end.
Rep rows 2–5 for crocodile st, ending with 2 tr bet next (skipped) 2-tr group.

NOTES
1) Cardigan is worked from bottom edge to yoke in one piece. Sleeves are worked directly onto the armhole down to the cuff.

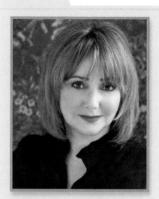

NICKY'S STORY
Nicky Epstein's unique, well-thought-out, and often quirky designs are instantly recognizable and have given life to over twenty books, including *Crocheting on the Edge* and *Crochet for Dolls*. After her gorgeous design for *Knit Red*, we couldn't wait to have her back for *Crochet Red*! It is important to Nicky to use her work to promote worthy causes. She has lost family and friends to heart disease and hopes to raise awareness of how serious a danger it is to women. It's hard to fit exercise and a healthy diet into Nicky's busy lifestyle—after all, she'd rather be sitting down to design or crochet! Living in New York, she gets in plenty of walking, especially when she knows she'll be sitting later. She also substitutes vegetable oils for animal fats, limits red meat and salt, and enjoys treats in moderation: stick to one piece of that antioxidant-rich dark chocolate!

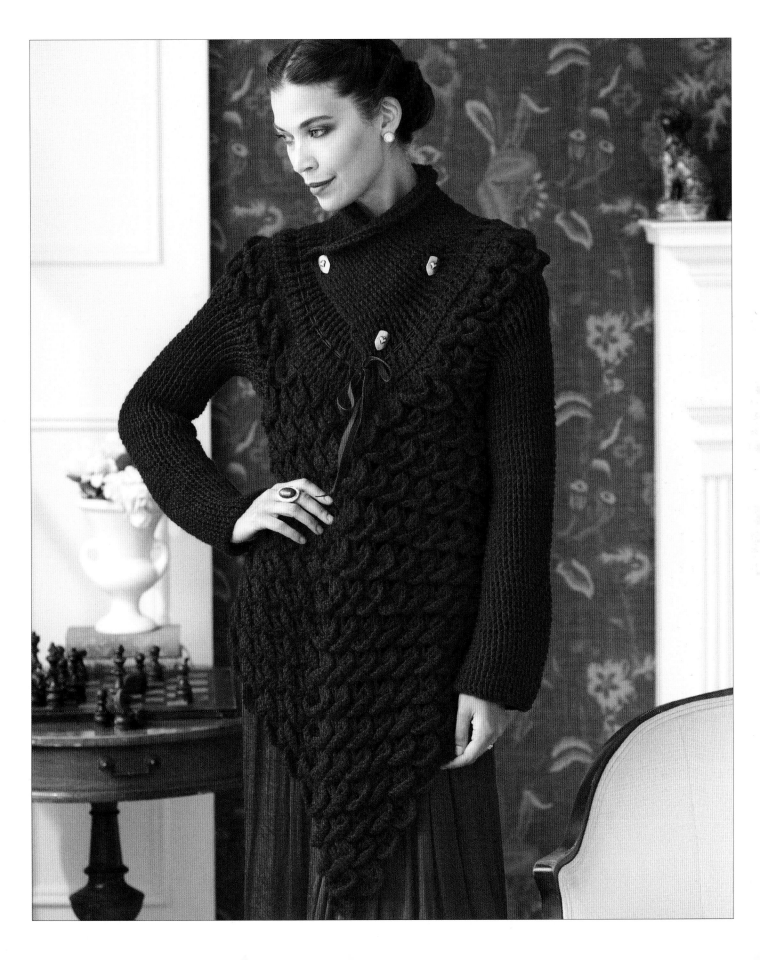

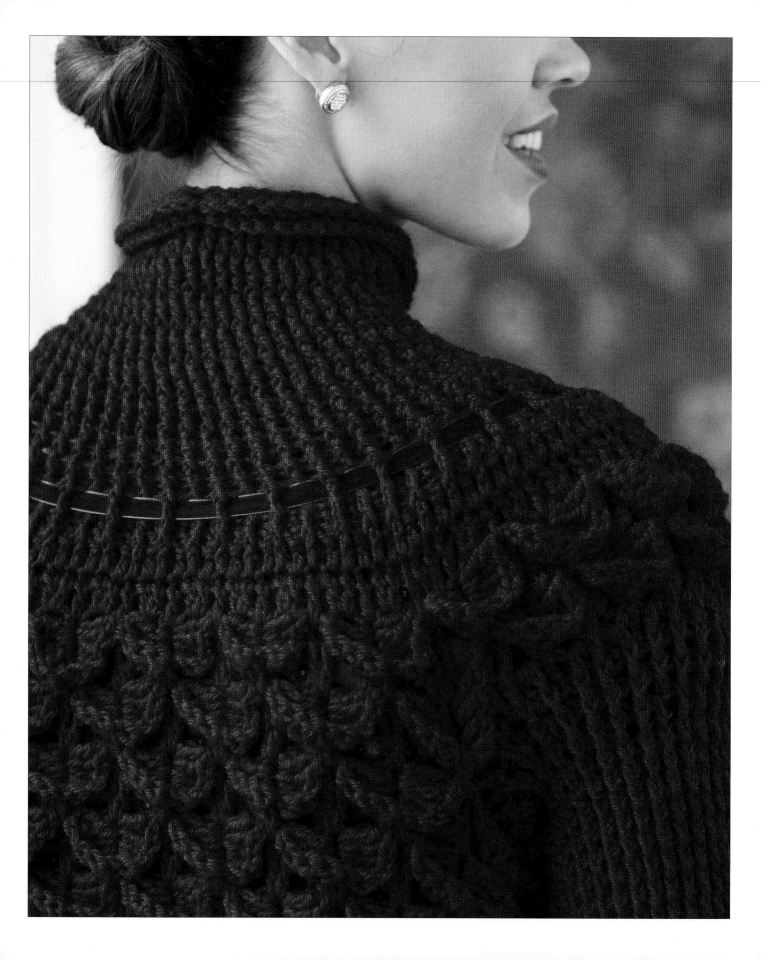

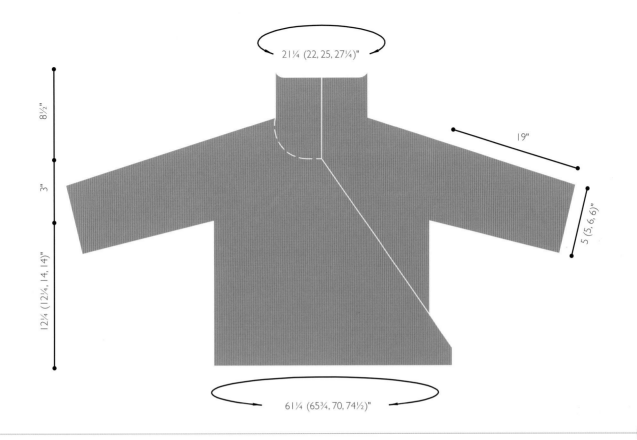

21¼ (22, 25, 27¼)"

8½"

19"

3"

5 (5, 6, 6)"

12¼ (12¼, 14, 14)"

61¼ (65¾, 70, 74½)"

2) When making 2-tr groups in crocodile stitch, place them into the 2-tr groups below—these are actually two rows below, the scales being worked on the intervening rows.

3) When making a 2-tr group that falls between two scales, ALSO work over the ch-2 between scales.

BODY

With larger hook, ch 172 (184, 196, 208).

Row 1 (RS) 2 tr in 4th ch from hook, *ch 2, sk 2 ch, 2 tr in next ch; rep from * to end— 57 (61, 65, 69) 2-tr groups.

Rows 2–9 (9, 11, 11) Rep rows 2–5 of crocodile st 2 (2, 3, 3) times—29 (31, 33, 35) scales on row 2.

Next 4 rows (all sizes) Rep rows 2–4 of crocodile st—6 (6, 8, 8) rows of scales.

FRONT PANEL SHAPING

Row 1 (RS) Ch 3, turn, sk first 2-tr group, *2 tr bet next 2-tr group (in center of scale), ch 2, 2 tr bet next 2-tr group (crochet bet last tr of next scale and first tr of prev scale and catching ch-2 bet scales), ch 2; rep from * to last (2) 2-tr groups, 2 tr bet next 2-tr group, leave rem 2-tr group unworked—55 (59, 63, 67) 2-tr groups.

Row 2 Ch 3, turn (turn work 90 degrees to crochet around prev tr on row below), *sk next 2-tr group, 5 tr around post of first tr of 2-tr group from top to base, ch 1, 5 tr around post of second tr of 2-tr group from base to top; rep from * to last 2-tr group, sk last 2-tr group—27 (29, 31, 33) scales.
Rep rows 1 and 2 six times more—21 (23, 25, 27) scales and 13 (13, 15, 15) rows of scales.

ARMHOLE SHAPING
AND YOKE

Row 1 (RS) Ch 3, turn, sk first 2-tr group, *2 tr bet next 2-tr group (in center of scale), ch 2, 2 tr bet next 2-tr group (crochet around last tr of next scale and first tr of prev scale), ch 2*; rep from * 4 (5, 5, 6) times more, fasten off. Sk 5 2-tr groups, join yarn w sl st to next tr group, ch 3, 2 tr bet same 2-tr group, rep from * to * 4 (4, 6, 6) times, fasten off. Sk 5 2-tr groups, join yarn with sl st to next tr group, ch 3, 2 tr bet same 2-tr group, rep from * to * 4 (5, 5, 6) times, 2 tr bet next 2-tr group, leave remaining 2-tr group unworked—31 (35, 39, 43) 2-tr groups.

Row 2 Ch 3, turn (turn work 90 degrees to crochet around prev tr on row below), *sk next 2-tr group, 5 tr around post of first tr of 2-tr group from top to base, ch 1, 5 tr around post of second tr of 2-tr group from

base to top*; rep from * across, **ch 47 (47, 53, 53) (armhole made), 5 tr around post of first tr of 2-tr group on back panel from top to base, ch 1, 5 tr around post of second tr of 2-tr group from base to top, rep from * to * across back panel; rep from ** to end, leave last 2-tr group unworked—16 (18, 20, 22) scales.

Row 3 Ch 3, turn, sk first 2-tr group, *2 tr bet next 2-tr group (in center of scale), ch 2, 2 tr bet next 2-tr group (crochet bet last tr of next scale and first tr of prev scale), ch 2*; rep from * to last 2 tr-group on front panel, 2 tr bet next 2-tr group, **ch 2, sk 2 ch, 2 tr in next ch; rep from ** to last 2 ch, ch 2, sk last 2 ch; rep from * across back panel and next armhole, rep from * to * across opposite panel to last 2 2-tr groups, 2 tr bet next 2-tr group, leave rem 2-tr group unworked—57 (61, 69, 73) 2-tr groups.

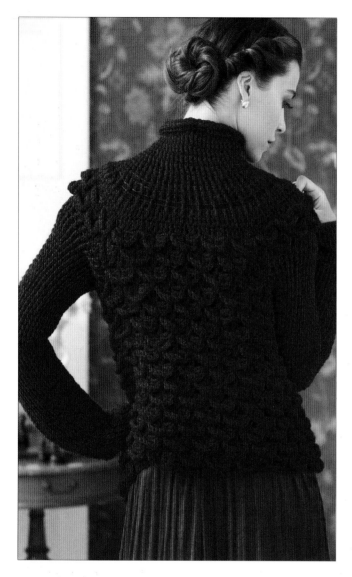

Row 4 Ch 3, turn (turn work 90 degrees to crochet around prev tr on row below), *sk next 2-tr group, 5 tr around post of first tr of 2-tr group from top to base, ch 1, 5 tr around post of second tr of 2-tr group from base to top; rep from * to last 2-tr group, sk last 2-tr group—29 (31, 35, 37) scales.
Rep rows 1 and 2 of front panel shaping—28 (30, 34, 36) scales.

COLLAR

Row 1 (RS) Change to smaller hook, ch 2, turn, (work in sts 1 row below), *dc bet next 2-tr group, 2 dc in next ch-2 sp; rep from * to last 2-tr group, dc bet next 2-tr group—169 (181, 205, 217) dc.
Row 2 Ch 3, turn, *FPtr around next dc, BPtr around next dc; rep from * to last dc, FPtr around next dc, tr in top of t-ch.
Row 3 Ch 3, turn, *BPtr around next tr, FPtr around next tr; rep from * to last tr, BPtr around next tr, tr in top of t-ch.
Row 4 Ch 3, turn, *FPtr around next tr, BPtr around next tr; rep from * to last tr, FPtr around next tr, tr in top of t-ch.
Row 5 Ch 2, turn, *BPdc around next tr, sk next tr; rep from * to last tr, BPdc around next tr, dc in top of t-ch—85 (91, 103, 109) dc.
Row 6 Ch 2, turn, FPdc around each dc across, dc in top of t-ch.
Row 7 Ch 2, turn, BPdc around each dc across, dc in top of t-ch.
Rep rows 6 and 7 eight times more. Fasten off.

SLEEVES

With smaller hook and RS facing, join yarn to underarm with sl st.
Rnd 1 (RS) Ch 2, 80 (80, 96, 96) dc evenly around armhole opening, by placing dc bet next 2-tr group, 2 dc in next ch-2 sp around, as much as possible. Do not join, place marker and move marker up with each rnd.
Rnd 2 *FPdc around next dc, BPdc around next dc; rep from * around.
Rnds 3 and 4 Rep rnd 2.
Rnd 5 *FPdc around next dc, sk next dc; rep from * around—40 (40, 48, 48) dc.
Rnd 6 FPdc around each dc across. Remove marker.
Rep rnd 6 until sleeve measures 19"/48.5cm, fasten off.

FINISHING

Block lightly to measurements. Using photo as guide, sew buttons to collar. Use spaces between stitches as buttonholes. Weave ribbon in and out of stitches on row 2 of collar; clip ends at an angle.❤

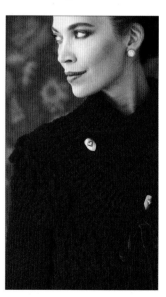

♥ NICKY'S TIP
GETTING 10 MINUTES OF ACTIVITY for every 60 minutes of sitting is important. Nicky suggests making exercise a mandatory requirement before starting a sedentary project.

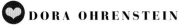

Floral Motif Wrap

Perfect your motif-making and joining skills with a lovely spring wrap. Floral motifs connect as you go to create a swirl of color and lace.

SIZE
Instructions are written for one size.

MEASUREMENTS
LENGTH 52"/132cm
WIDTH 18"/45.5cm

MATERIALS
• 2 3½oz/100g hanks (each approx 420yd/384m) of Madelinetosh *Tosh Merino Light* (superwash merino) in wilted rose (1)
• Size C/2 (2.75mm) crochet hook *or size to obtain gauge*
• Tapestry needle

GAUGE
Large motif = 6"/15cm from point diagonally across to opposite point using size C/2 (2.75mm) crochet hook.
➤Take time to check gauge.

STITCH GLOSSARY
popcorn Work 5 dc in specified st, remove hook from work, leaving lp loose, insert hook in first dc of this group and draw loose lp through.

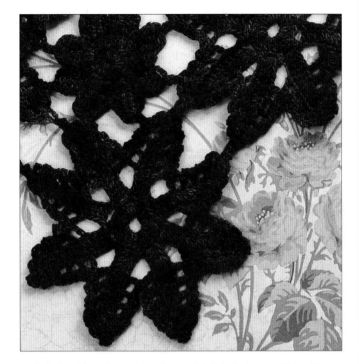

dtr3tog (double treble crochet 3 together) *[Yo 3 times, insert hook in next st and draw up a lp (5 lps on hook), yo and draw through 2 lps on hook] 3 times; rep from * 2 times more, yo and draw through all 4 lps on hook.

NOTES
1) In rnd 3 of large petal motif, when working into the base of ch, make sure to line up dcs with the 4th, 6th, and 8th of the petal sts. The base chain can be tricky to read. The dcs should be symmetrical on right and left sides of each petal.
2) In last rnd of large petal motif, the ch-5 points may appear to be slightly left of center. This will even out when the motifs are joined and the wrap is blocked.
3) When joining motifs, make sure they all have RS facing. Refer to assembly diagram as you join motifs.
4) To make a wider wrap, work additional vertical rows of large petal motifs and fill in the smaller motifs in established pat. To make a longer wrap, work an additional horizontal row of large petal motifs and fill in with smaller motifs in established pat, alternating between daisy motifs and popcorn flowers as you work across.

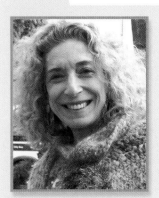

DORA'S STORY
Dora Ohrenstein is the creative genius behind *Crochet Insider*, an online resource for news, techniques, designer interviews, and patterns. She teaches online classes on everything from sweater shaping to designing, including one with fellow *Crochet Red* designer Charles Voth. Manhattanite Dora finds inspiration in fashion trends—window shopping is one of her favorite pastimes! Dora is also a trained singer who toured for ten years with the Philip Glass Ensemble and still gives singing lessons when she's not designing. Dora feels lucky that her family has not been personally affected by heart disease, and she joined the Stitch Red campaign to help raise awareness so other families, regardless of their history, can lessen their chances of a run-in with heart disease. To maintain her own health, she practices yoga regularly and eats a fresh salad every evening, dressed with heart-healthy extra virgin olive oil and balsamic vinegar.

WRAP

LARGE PETAL MOTIF A

Note This motif is not connected to other motifs.

Make an adjustable ring.

Rnd 1 (RS) Ch 3 (counts as first dc), work 23 dc in ring; join with sl st in top of beg ch-3—24 dc.

Rnd 2 (petal rnd) Ch 1, sc in same st as joining, *ch 12 (petal foundation ch made), working in back lps (BL) of petal foundation ch, sc BL in 2nd ch from hook, sc BL in next ch, hdc BL in next 2 ch, dc BL in next 7 ch, sk next 2 dc of rnd 1**, sc in next dc (petal made); rep from * 7 times more, ending last rep at **; join with sl st in first sc—8 petals.

Rnd 3 Working in front lps (FL) of petal foundation ch, sl st over next 4 ch, ch 4 (counts as dc, ch 1), *sk next ch, [dc FL in next ch, ch 1, sk next ch] 3 times; cont around tip and working in sts down other side of same petal, (dc, ch 1, dc) in ch-1 sp at tip of petal, ch 1, dc in 2nd sc, ch 1, sk next hdc, dc in next hdc, [ch 1, sk next dc, dc in next dc] twice**, dc FL in 4th ch of next petal foundation ch, ch 1; rep from * 7 times more, ending last rep at **; join with sl st in 3rd ch of beg ch-4.

Rnd 4 Ch 1, sc in first ch-1 sp, *[ch 3, sc in next ch-1 sp] 4 times, ch 5, sc in same ch-1 sp, [ch 3, sc in next ch-1 sp] 4 times**, sc in first ch-1 sp of next petal; rep from * 7 times more, ending last rep at **; join with sl st in first sc. Fasten off.

LARGE PETAL MOTIF B

Note This motif is connected at 2 points to 1 previous motif.

Work same as large petal motif A through rnd 3.

Rnd 4 (joining rnd) Ch 1, sc in first ch-1 sp, *[ch 3, sc in next ch-1 sp] 4 times, ch 5, sc in same ch-1 sp, [ch 3, sc in next ch-1 sp] 4 times, sc in first ch-1 sp of next petal; rep from * 5 times more, [ch 3, sc in next ch-1 sp] 4 times, ch 2, sl st in ch-5 sp at point of large petal motif A, ch 2, sc in same ch-1 sp of large petal motif B, [ch 3, sc in next ch-1 sp] 4 times, sc in first ch-1 sp of last petal, [ch 3, sc in next ch-1 sp] 4 times, ch 2, sl st in ch-5 sp at next point of large petal motif A, ch 2, sc in same ch-1 sp of large petal motif B, [ch 3, sc in next ch-1 sp] 4 times; join with sl st in first sc. Fasten off.

LARGE PETAL MOTIF C

Work same as large petal motif B, joining to two points on large petal motif A as shown on assembly diagram.

LARGE PETAL MOTIF D

Note This motif is connected at 2 points to each of 2 previous motifs.

Work same as large petal motif A through rnd 3. Refer to assembly diagram for points on large petal motifs B and C to which this motif is to be joined.

Rnd 4 (joining rnd) Ch 1, sc in first ch-1 sp, *[ch 3, sc in next ch-1 sp] 4 times, ch 5, sc in same ch-1 sp, [ch 3, sc in next ch-1 sp] 4 times, sc in first ch-1 sp of next petal; rep from * 3 times more, [ch 3, sc in next ch-1 sp] 4 times, ch 2, sl st in ch-5 sp at point of large petal motif B, ch 2, sc in same ch-1 sp of large petal motif D, [ch 3, sc in next ch-1 sp] 4 times, sc in first ch-1 sp of next petal, [ch 3, sc in next ch-1 sp] 4 times, ch 2, sl st in ch-5 sp at next point of large petal motif B, ch 2, sc in same ch-1 sp of large petal motif D, [ch 3, sc in next ch-1 sp] 4 times, sc in first ch-1 sp of next petal, [ch 3, sc in next ch-1 sp] 4 times, ch 2, sl st in ch-5 sp at point of large petal motif C, ch 2, sc in same ch-1 sp of large petal motif D, [ch 3, sc in next ch-1 sp] 4 times, sc in first ch-1 sp of last petal, [ch 3, sc in next ch-1 sp] 4 times, ch 2, sl st in ch-5 sp at next point of large petal motif C, ch 2, sc in same ch-1 sp of large petal motif D, [ch 3, sc in next ch-1 sp] 4 times; join with sl st in first sc. Fasten off.

DAISY MOTIF

Make an adjustable ring.

Rnd 1 Ch 3 (counts as first dc here and throughout), work 15 dc in ring; join with sl st in top of beg ch-3—16 dc.

Rnd 2 Ch 3, 3 dc in same st as joining, *sk next dc, 4 dc in next dc; rep from * to last dc, sk last dc; join with sl st in top of beg ch-3—32 dc.

Rnd 3 Ch 1, sc in same st as joining, *ch 5, dtr3tog over next 3 dc, ch 2, sl st in ch-3 sp of large petal motif (see assembly diagram), ch 2, sl st in top of dtr3tog just made, ch 5, sc in next dc; rep from * around, connecting to points on large petal motifs A, B, C, and D as shown in assembly diagram; join with sl st in first sc—8 petals. Fasten off.

LARGE PETAL MOTIF E

Make another large petal motif and connect it to large petal motif C the same way large petal motif C was connected to large petal motif A.

LARGE PETAL MOTIF F

Make another large petal motif and connect it to large petal motifs D and E the same way large petal motif D was connected to large petal motifs B and C.

Make another daisy motif and connect it to the 8 points around the outer edge of the opening between large petal motifs C, D, E, and F. You should now have 2 vertical rows consisting of 3 large petal motifs, and one vertical row of 2 daisy motifs.

LARGE PETAL MOTIF G

Make another large petal motif and connect it to large petal motif B the same way large petal motif B was connected to large petal motif A.

LARGE PETAL MOTIF H

Work another large petal motif and connect it to large petal motifs D and G the same way large petal motif D was connected to large petal motifs B and C.

POPCORN FLOWER

Ch 3.

Rnd 1 Work 8 sc in 2nd ch from hook; join with sl st in first sc—8 sc.

Rnd 2 Ch 1, 2 sc in each sc around; join with sl st in first sc—16 sc.

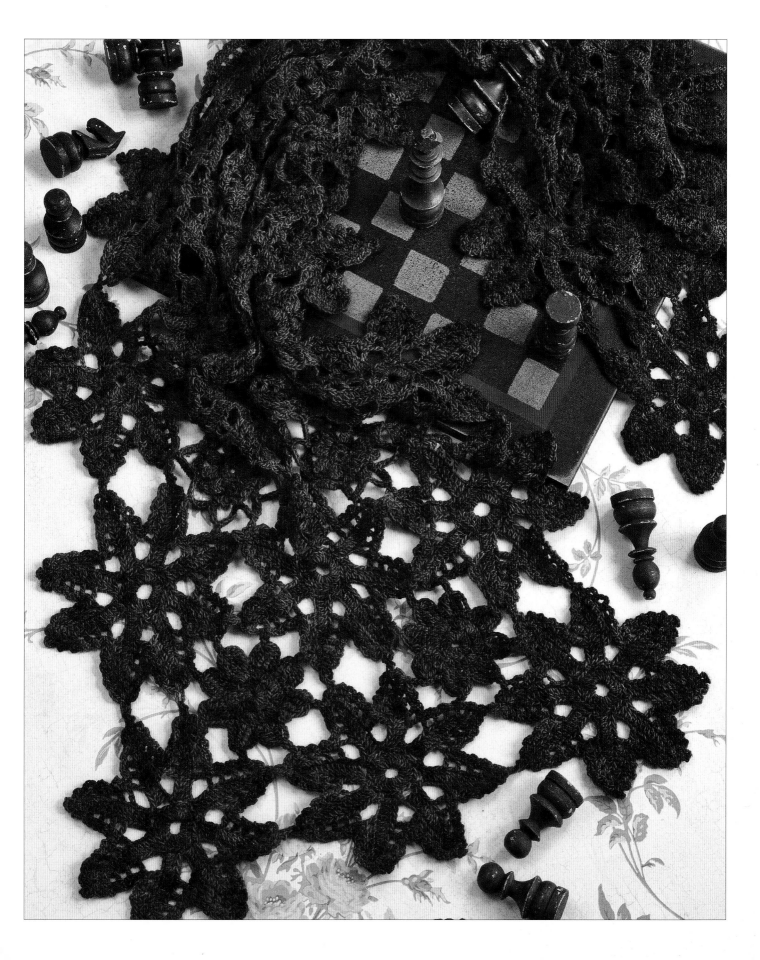

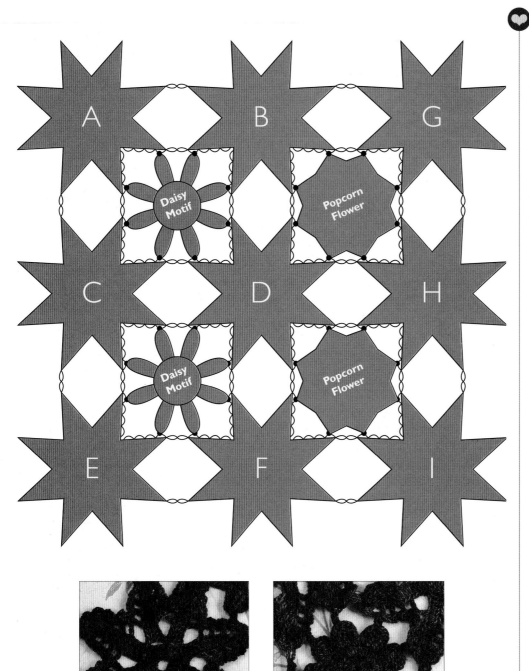

Rnd 3 Ch 3, popcorn in first sc (using beg ch-3 as first dc of popcorn), *ch 6, sl st in 4th ch from hook (picot made), ch 2**, sk next sc, popcorn in next sc; rep from * around, ending last rep at **, sk last sc; join with sl st in top of first popcorn—8 popcorns.

Rnd 4 Ch 1, sc in same st as joining, *ch 9, sc in top of next popcorn; rep from * around; join with sl st in first sc—8 ch-9 sps and 8 sc.

Note In next rnd, connect popcorn flower to the 8 ch-3 sps around the outer edge of the opening between large petal motifs B, D, H, and G.

Rnd 5 Ch 1, *5 sc in next ch-9 sp, sc in ch-3 sp of large petal motif, 5 sc in same ch-9 sp; rep from * around; join with sl st in first sc. Fasten off.

LARGE PETAL MOTIF I
Make another large petal motif and connect it to large petal motifs H and F the same way large petal motif D was connected to large petal motifs B and C.

Make another popcorn flower and connect it to the 8 ch-3 sps around the outer edge of the opening between large petal motifs D, F, I, and H. You should now have 3 vertical rows each consisting of 3 large petal motifs, one vertical row of 2 daisy motifs, and one vertical row of 2 popcorn flowers.

Continue making and joining motifs in the same manner until there are a total of 8 vertical rows of large petal motifs, 4 vertical rows of daisy motifs, and 3 vertical rows of popcorn flowers.

FINISHING
Block lightly to measurements.♥

DEBORAH NEWTON

Oversized Lacy Pullover

Light and airy but heavy on style, this swingy, loose-fitting sweater with cutouts and lace spans the seasons.

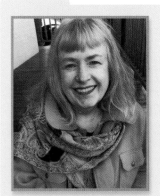

SIZES
Instructions are written for size Small. Changes for Medium and Large are in parentheses. (Shown in size Small.)

MEASUREMENTS
BUST 44 (48, 54)"/111.5 (122, 137)cm
LENGTH
25 (26, 27)"/63.5 (66, 68.5)cm
UPPER ARM CIRCUMFERENCE
20 (22, 24)"/51 (56, 61)cm

MATERIALS
• 8 (9, 10) .88oz/25g hanks (each approx 330yd/302m) of Shibui Knits *Silk Cloud* (mohair/silk) in #2031 poppy **1**
• Size 7 (4.5mm) crochet hook *or size to obtain gauge*
• Tapestry needle

GAUGES
1 square motif = 4"/10cm × 4"/10cm with 2 strands held together using size 7 (4.5mm) crochet hook.
4 shells and 10 rows = 4"/10cm × 4¼"/11cm over scallop pat with 2 strands held together using size 7 (4.5mm) crochet hook.
➤Take time to check gauges.

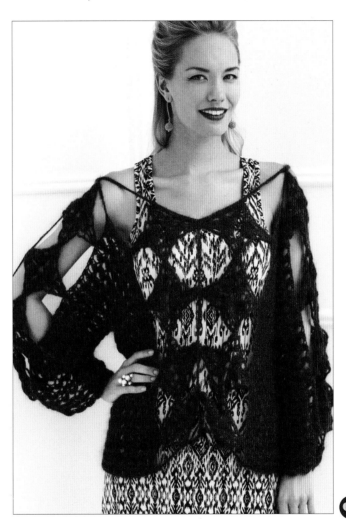

STITCH GLOSSARY
dc5tog (double crochet 5 together) *Yo, insert hook in indicated st and draw up a loop, yo and draw through 2 loops on hook; rep from * 4 times more in next indicated st, yo and draw through all 6 loops on hook.

dc6tog (double crochet 6 together) *Yo, insert hook in indicated st and draw up a loop, yo and draw through 2 loops on hook; rep from * 5 times more in next indicated st, yo and draw through all 7 loops on hook.

DEBORAH'S STORY
Rhode Island native Deborah Newton has been creating knit and crochet fashions for over thirty years. Her designs appear regularly in the top magazines, and she's authored several books, including *Finishing School.* A longtime knitter, Deborah taught herself to crochet to indulge her fascination with the unique look and feel of crocheted fabrics. When she's not creating fiber art with needles, hooks, and yarn, Deborah loves to swim in the nearby Atlantic and is an enthusiastic gardener. Her cocker spaniel, Brownie, helps her stay active, too—he's always ready for a walk about town! Deborah won't soon forget seeing her mother go through a heart valve replacement, and that experience stands as a daily reminder to take care of her own heart. She practices yoga every day, and doesn't drive a car in favor of walking where she needs to go.

DEBORAH'S TIP
GARDENING IS GREAT EXERCISE, and also gives Deborah fresh, yummy vegetables to create healthy homemade salads!

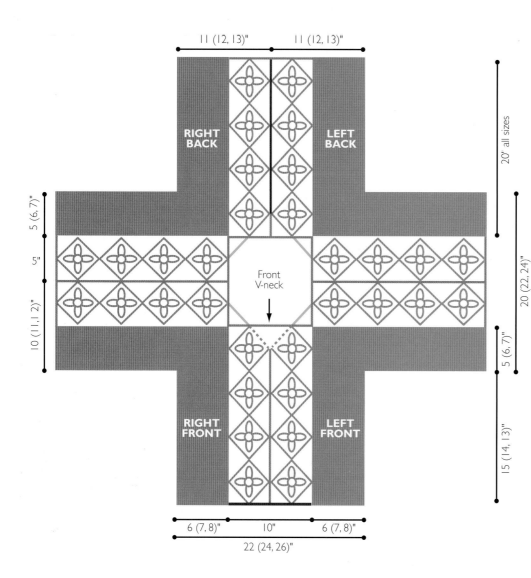

11 (12, 13)" **11 (12, 13)"**

RIGHT BACK

LEFT BACK

20" all sizes

5 (6, 7)"

5"

Front V-neck

10 (11, 12)"

20 (22, 24)"

5 (6, 7)"

RIGHT FRONT

LEFT FRONT

15 (14, 13)"

6 (7, 8)" 10" 6 (7, 8)"

22 (24, 26)"

ch 2, dc) in next dc, dc in next 2 dc, ch 2, (3 dc, ch 5, 3 dc) in ch-9 sp, ch 2**; dc in next 2 dc; rep from * around, ending at **, sl st in top of beg ch—48 dc.

Rnd 3 Ch 2, dc5tog over next 5 dc (sk ch-2 sp), *ch 5, sk 1 dc, dc in next dc, ch 3, (2 dc, ch 2, 2 dc) in ch-5 sp, ch 3, sk 1 dc, dc in next dc, ch 5**, dc6tog over next 6 sc (sk ch-2 sp); rep from * around, ending at **, sl st to top of dc5tog.

Rnd 4 Ch 1, *5 sc in ch-5 sp, sc in next dc, 3 sc in ch-3 sp, sc in next 2 dc, 2 dc in ch-2 sp, sc in next 2 dc, 3 sc in ch-3 sp, sc in next dc, 5 sc in ch-5 sp, sc in dctog; rep from * around, sl st to first sc, fasten off.

LEFT PANEL (MAKE 2)
Ch 137.
Row 1 Dc in 4th ch from hook, *ch 2, sk 6 ch, (dc, ch 3, dc) in next ch (v-st made); rep from * to last 7 ch, ch 2, sk 6 ch, (dc, ch 1, dc) in last ch—18 v-sts.
Work rows 2 and 3 of scallop pat 7 (8, 9) times.

SLEEVE
Row 1 Ch 3, turn, 4 dc in ch-1 sp, 8 dc in next 4 (5, 6) ch-3 sps, 5 dc in next ch-3 sp, leave remaining sts unworked—4 (5, 6) shells.
Rep row 3 of scallop pat once, then rows 2 and 3 fourteen times, then row 2 once more. Fasten off.

RIGHT PANEL (MAKE 2)
Ch 137.
Row 1 Dc in 4th ch from hook, *ch 2, sk 6 ch, (dc, ch 3, dc) in next ch (v-st made); rep from * to last 7 ch, ch 2, sk 6 ch, (dc, ch 1, dc) in last ch—18 v-sts.
Work rows 2 and 3 of scallop pat 6 (7, 8) times, then row 2 once more.

COLOR KEY
A
B
C
D

SCALLOP PATTERN
Chain a multiple of 7 plus 4.
Row 1 (WS) Dc in 4th ch from hook, *ch 2, sk 6 ch, (dc, ch 3, dc) in next ch; rep from * to last 7 ch, ch 2, sk 6 ch, (dc, ch 1, dc) in last ch.
Row 2 Ch 3, turn, 4 dc in ch-1 sp, 8 dc in each ch-3 sp across to t-ch (shell made), 5 dc in t-ch sp.
Row 3 Ch 4, turn, dc in first dc, *ch 2, sk 7 dc, (dc, ch 3, dc) in next dc; rep from * to last shell, ch 2, (dc, ch 1, dc) in top of t-ch.
Rep rows 2 and 3 for scallop pat.

NOTES
1) Two strands of yarn are held together throughout.
2) Sweater is designed to have an oversized fit.

SQUARE MOTIF (MAKE 32)
Ch 10, join with sl st in first ch to form a ring.
Rnd 1 (RS) Ch 3 (counts as dc), 4 dc in ring, [ch 9, 5 dc in ring] 3 times, ch 9, join with sl st to top of beg ch—20 dc.
Rnd 2 Ch 3, dc in next dc, *(dc,

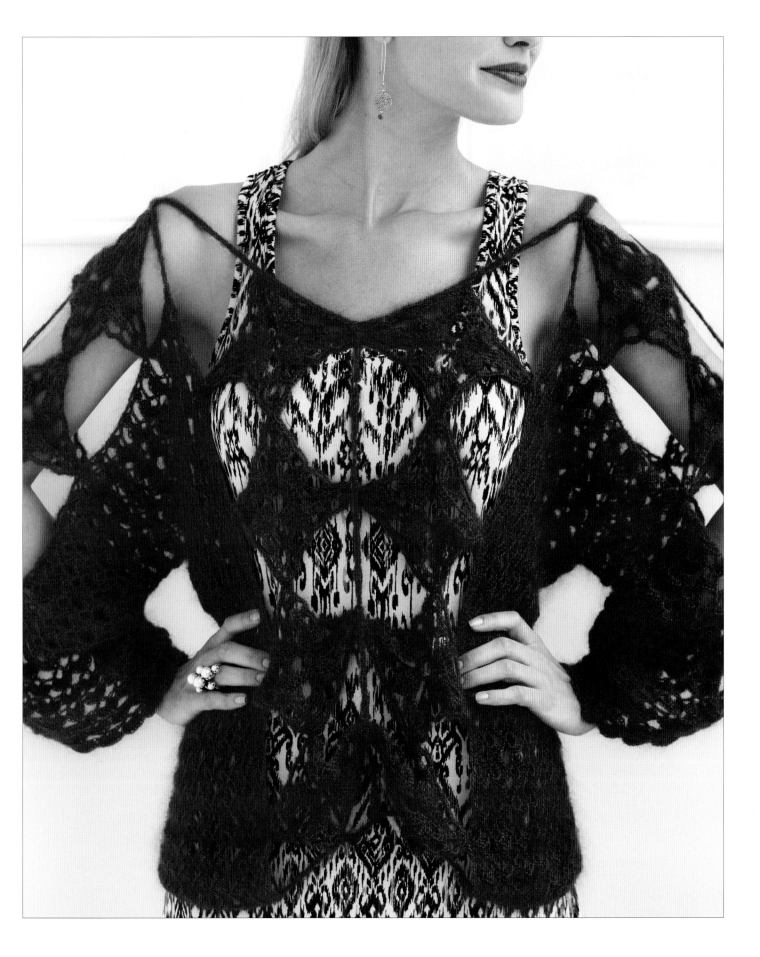

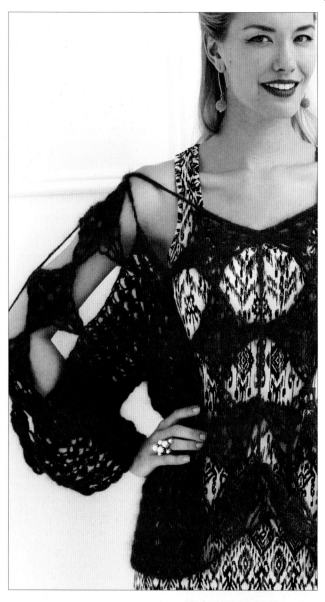

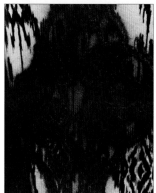

SLEEVE

Row 1 Ch 4, turn, dc in first dc, *ch 2, sk 7 dc, (dc, ch 3, dc) in next dc; rep from * 3 (4, 5) times more, ch 2, sk 7 dc, (dc, ch 1, dc) in next dc, leave remaining sts unworked.
Work rows 2 and 3 of scallop pat 15 times, then row 2 once more. Fasten off.

FINISHING

Block motifs and panels to schematic measurements. Pin right and left panels together with right sides facing. With tapestry needle, whipstitch underarm seam together. Join a double strand of yarn to underarm with sl st, *ch 3, sl st to center of v-st and shell at same time; rep from * to lower edge, fasten off. Rep on opposite set of panels.

JOINING MOTIFS

Using tapestry needle, sew 8 motifs together (2 rows of 4 motifs each) at each corner point. Sew one set of 8 motifs to between right and left front panels at each corner point. Rep between right and left back panels, right sleeve panels, and left sleeve panels. See schematic for location of motifs.

STABILIZING CHAINS

"A" chain Join a double strand to lower corner of left front panel with sl st, ch 10, sl st in corner point of next motif, ch 20, sl st in corner point of next motif, ch 10, sl st to lower corner of right front panel. Turn, sl st in each ch and sl st across, fasten off. Rep on lower and upper edge of back panel and lower and upper edge of both sleeves. See schematic for location of "A" chain lines.
"B" chain Turn sweater inside out with WS facing. Join double strand of yarn to center of "A" chain on lower back edge with sl st, ch 10, *sl st to corner point of next motif, ch 20; rep from * 2 times more, sl st to corner point of last motif, ch 10, sl st to center of "A" chain on upper back edge. Turn, sl st in each ch and sl st across, fasten off. Rep on each sleeve. See schematic for location of "B" chain line.
Front chain Join double strand of yarn to center of "A" chain on lower front edge with sl st, ch 10, *sl st to corner point of next motif, ch 20; rep from * 2 times more, sl st to corner point of last motif. Turn, sl st in each ch and sl st across, fasten off. See schematic for location of front chain line.
Neckline edge Turn sweater right side out. Join a double strand to front of V-neck with sl st, sl st in each st across motif ("D" line on schematic), *ch 20 ("C" line on schematic), sl st to next corner point of motif on sleeve, sc in each sl st across "A" line to next motif at corner point; rep on back edge and opposite sleeve edge, ch 20, sl st to next corner point of motif on front, sl st in each st across motif.
Next rnd Sk first sl st, sc in each st around neck to last 2 sts, sc in next st, sl st to first sc. Fasten off. ❤

♥ ROBYN CHACHULA

Flower Garland Cowl

This uniquely striking but easy-to-crochet accessory is composed of beautiful oversized tulipe motifs joined into a drapey floral garland.

■■□□

SIZE
Instructions are written for one size.

MEASUREMENTS
CIRCUMFERENCE
30"/76cm
HEIGHT
8"/20.5 cm

MATERIALS
• 2 3½oz/100g hanks (each approx 205yd/187m) of Lorna's Laces *Lion and Lamb* (wool/silk) in Ysolda red (④)
• Size I/9 (5.5mm) crochet hook *or size to obtain gauge*
• Tapestry needle

GAUGE
Tulipe motif = 5"/12.5cm in diameter using size I/9 (5.5mm) crochet hook.
➤ Take time to check gauge.

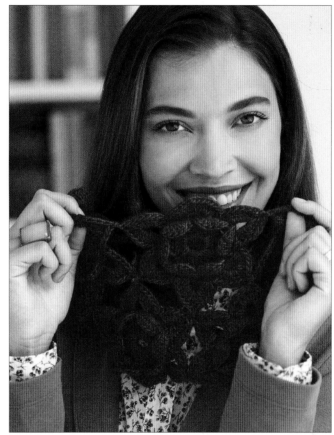

STITCH GLOSSARY
Ch 2 join Sl st in adjoining ch-2 sp on adjacent motif, ch 1.

NOTES
1) Ch-3 counts as 1 dc throughout.
2) Completed cowl will have 2 rows of 6 motifs each.

COWL
TULIPE MOTIF (MAKE 11)
Ch 8, sl st into first ch to form ring.
Rnd 1 (RS) Ch 3 (counts as 1 dc), 23 dc in ring, join rnd with sl st in top of beg-ch, do not turn—24 dc.
Rnd 2 Ch 1, sc in top of beg-ch, *ch 3, sk 1 dc, sc in next dc; rep from * to last 2 dc, ch 1, hdc in first sc (counts as a ch-3 sp), do not turn—12 ch-3 sps.

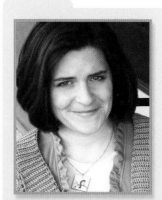

ROBYN'S STORY
It might surprise you that crochet superstar Robyn Chachula started her career as a structural engineer. While that may not seem related to crochet design, the two pursuits have elements in common: visualization, careful planning, and attacking a project one piece at a time while fulfilling a larger vision. Robyn's mother taught her to crochet over ten years ago, and she devoured every book she could find on the subject, starting with granny squares and moving up from there. Now, with several books to her name, along with numerous patterns and instructional DVDs, Robyn is known as the mother of crochet schematics and diagrams. Her *Blueprint Crochet* series revolutionized patterns by giving crocheters a visual step-by-step guide to each stitch. With a family history of stroke, Robyn takes special care of her health by exercising daily, combining yoga and trail jogging to get in both cardio and strength training.

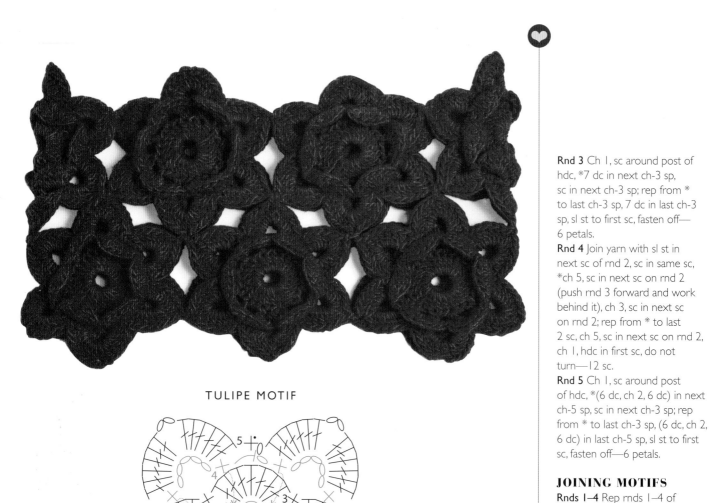

TULIPE MOTIF

Rnd 3 Ch 1, sc around post of hdc, *7 dc in next ch-3 sp, sc in next ch-3 sp; rep from * to last ch-3 sp, 7 dc in last ch-3 sp, sl st to first sc, fasten off— 6 petals.

Rnd 4 Join yarn with sl st in next sc of rnd 2, sc in same sc, *ch 5, sc in next sc on rnd 2 (push rnd 3 forward and work behind it), ch 3, sc in next sc on rnd 2; rep from * to last 2 sc, ch 5, sc in next sc on rnd 2, ch 1, hdc in first sc, do not turn—12 sc.

Rnd 5 Ch 1, sc around post of hdc, *(6 dc, ch 2, 6 dc) in next ch-5 sp, sc in next ch-3 sp; rep from * to last ch-3 sp, (6 dc, ch 2, 6 dc) in last ch-5 sp, sl st to first sc, fasten off—6 petals.

JOINING MOTIFS
Rnds 1–4 Rep rnds 1–4 of tulipe motif.
Rnd 5 Rep rnd 5 of tulipe motif, substituting "ch 2, join" for "ch 2" when motifs are adjacent.
Note In first row, motifs are joined at 2 petals; in second row, motifs are joined at 4 petals. See photo as a guide for placement.

FINISHING
Block lightly to measurements.♥

STITCH KEY

- sl st
- ch
+ sc
⊤ hdc
† dc
✕ attach with sl st

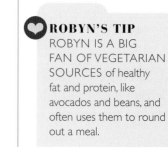

ROBYN'S TIP
ROBYN IS A BIG FAN OF VEGETARIAN SOURCES of healthy fat and protein, like avocados and beans, and often uses them to round out a meal.

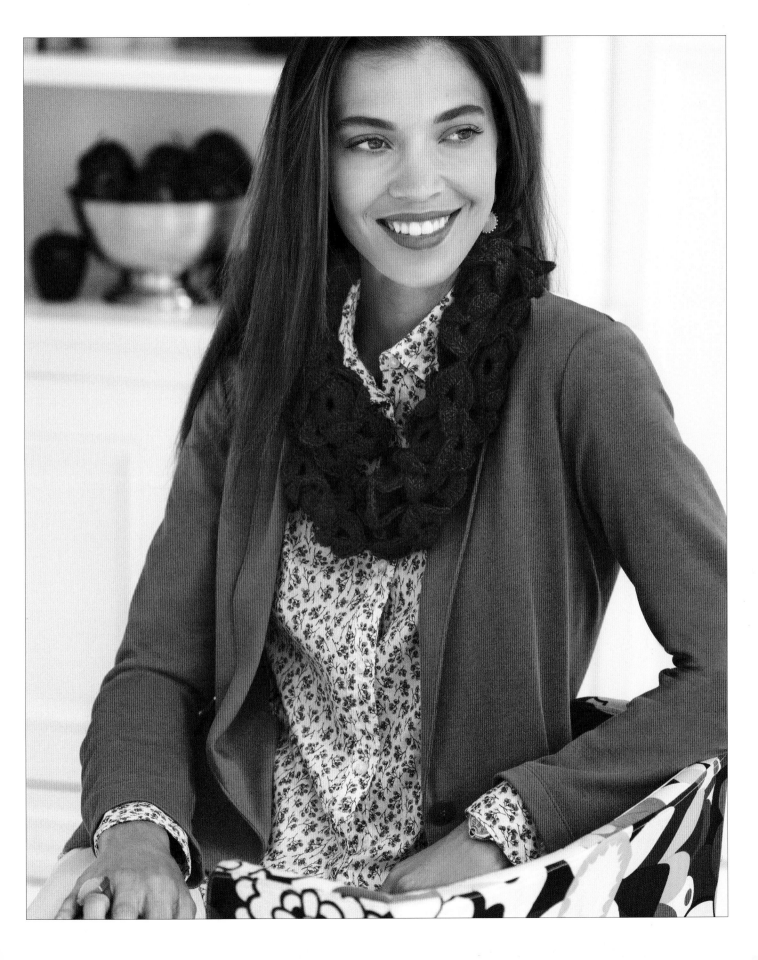

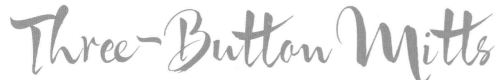

Three-Button Mitts

With straightforward shaping, an easy stitch pattern based on single crochet, and a chance to show off your favorite buttons, these mitts are a joy to make and wear.

■■□□

SIZE
Instructions are written for one size.

MEASUREMENTS
PALM CIRCUMFERENCE
6"/15cm

LENGTH 7"/18cm

MATERIALS
• 1 1¾oz/50g hank (each approx 196yd/180m) of Hand Maiden Fine Yarns *Swiss Mountain Cashmere and Silk* (cashmere/silk) in vermillion **①**

• Size D/3 (3.25mm) crochet hook *or size to obtain gauge*

• Locking stitch markers

• Tapestry needle

• 6 buttons, approx ⅜"/1cm diameter

GAUGE
28 sc and 32 rows = 4"/10cm over sc stitch pattern using size D/3 (3.25mm) crochet hook.
➤ Take time to check gauge.

NOTE
Stitch pattern is reversible, so a marked side is specified to aid in assembly later (leave marker in until assembly is complete). One mitt will be worn with unmarked side out, the other with marked side out; seam and sew buttons to tabs accordingly.

LEFT MITT
BUTTON TAB
Ch 17.
Row 1 2 sc in back bump of 3rd ch from hook, *sk 1 ch, 2 sc in back bump of next ch; rep from * to end—16 sc.
Rows 2–6 Ch 2, *sk 1 sc, 2 sc in next sc; rep from * to end.

WRIST
Row 1 Ch 2, *sk 1 sc, 2 sc in next sc; rep from * to end.
Place a locking marker into work on side facing you to aid in assembly later.
Row 2 Ch 33, 2 sc in back bump of 3rd ch from hook, *sk 1 ch, 2 sc in back bump of next ch; rep from * to button tab sts, **sk 1 sc, 2 sc in next sc; rep from ** to end—48 sc.
Row 3 Ch 2, *sk 1 sc, 2 sc in next sc; rep from * to end—48 sc.
Rep row 3 until work measures 3"/7.5cm (not including button tab), ending after an unmarked-side row.

THUMB GUSSET
Place locking markers in 26th and 36th sc.
Row 1 Ch 2, *sk 1 sc, 2 sc in next sc; rep from * ending with 2 sc in first marked sc, *turn*—26 sc.
Row 2 Ch 2, *sk 1 sc, 2 sc in next sc; rep from * 12 times more—26 sc.
Rep row 2 twice more.

HAND
Row 1 (marked side) Ch 2, *sk 1 sc, 2 sc in next sc; rep from * 12 times more, ch 8 loosely, 2 sc in next marked st, **sk 1 sc, 2 sc in next sc; rep from ** to end—14 sc after thumb opening.
Row 2 Ch 2, [sk 1 sc, 2 sc in next sc] 7 times, [sk 1 ch, 2 sc in back bump of next ch] 4 times, [sk 1 sc, 2 sc in next sc] 13 times—48 sc.
Row 3 Ch 2, *sk 1 sc, 2 sc in next sc; rep from * to end—48 sc.
Rep row 3 until work measures just shy of 3"/7.5cm from thumb opening, ending after an unmarked-side row.
Button loop row (marked side)
Ch 2, sk 1 sc, 2 sc in next sc, *ch 2, [sk 1 sc, 2 sc in next sc] 3 times; rep from * once more, ch 2, **sk 1 sc, 2 sc in next sc, rep from ** to end.
Fasten off, leaving an 18"/46cm tail for seaming.

FINISHING
Block piece lightly to measurements. Fold in half, marked sides together. Join edges with mattress stitch as follows: insert needle just inside chain edges, under 2 sc on ending edge and under 2 strands on beginning edge, until you reach button tab on one side and third button loop on the other. Take an extra stitch to strengthen. Tuck button tab to inside and whipstitch short edge down.
Sc evenly around thumb opening. Fasten off.
Sew buttons on button tabs opposite button loops.

RIGHT MITT
Work as for left mitt up to finishing. For seaming, fold with *unmarked* sides together. Complete as for left mitt.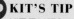

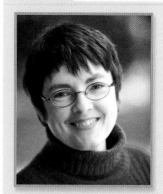

KIT'S STORY
When Kit Hutchin opened Churchmouse Yarns & Teas on Bainbridge Island near Seattle, she finally merged her two loves: yarn and fine teas. She has created her own designs under the Churchmouse label, including a few tea cozies! Kit has ties to heart disease—she lost her mom to a stroke, and a dear friend and a staff member to heart attacks—but what really made her want to contribute to *Crochet Red* was learning that more women die from heart disease than from any other killer. She immediately changed some unhealthy habits, including a propensity to sit (and knit or crochet) too long. Now she carries projects with her and works as she walks! She even stitches while her husband golfs, a form of exercise they call "knolfing." Kit starts each day with a healthy, sustaining bowl of oatmeal and a cup of antioxidant-rich tea.

♥ KIT'S TIP
KIT TAKES ADVANTAGE OF LOCAL FARMER'S MARKETS to source the freshest produce for her cooking, along with the heart-healthy salmon available year-round in her region.

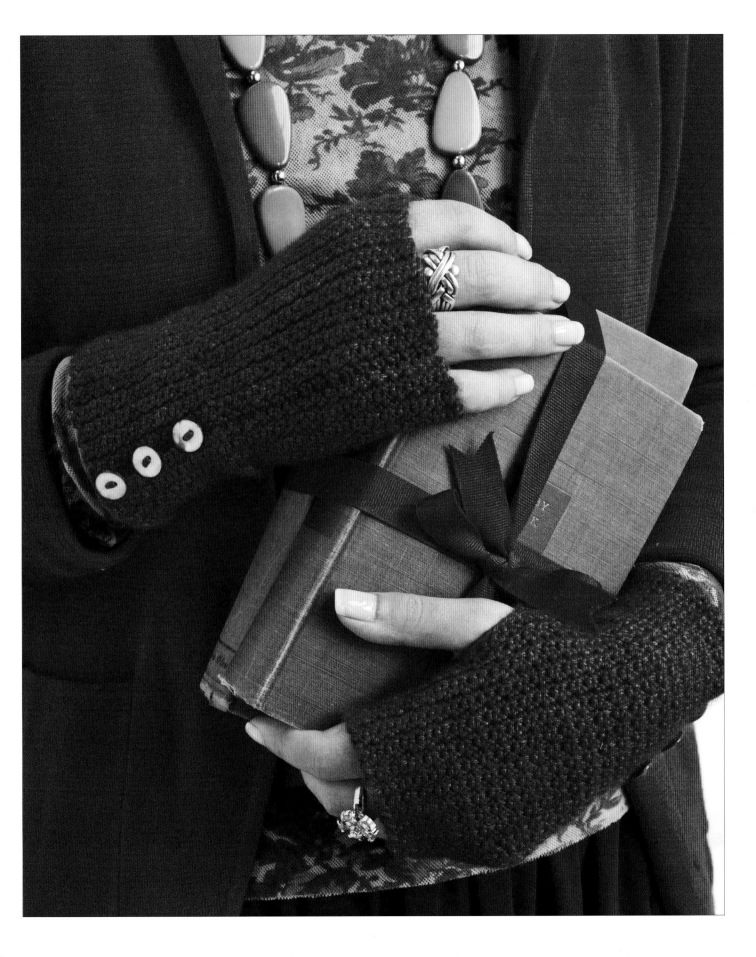

Reversible Wrap

A warm woolen wrap gets modern style from tonal stripes and a seam down the center back that serves as a design element.

■■□□

SIZE
Instructions are written for one size.

MEASUREMENTS
WIDTH 22"/56cm
LENGTH 70" long/178cm

MATERIALS
• 8 1¾oz/50g balls
(each approx 122yd/112m)
of Classic Elite *Liberty Wool*
(superwash wool) each
in #7855 raspberry red (A)
and #7827 wine (B) **④**
• Size 7 (4.5mm) crochet hook
or size to obtain gauge
• Tapestry needle

GAUGE
3 shells and 11 rows =
5¼"/15.5cm and 4"/10cm
over reversible shell st pat using
size 7 (4.5mm) crochet hook.
➤Take time to check gauge.

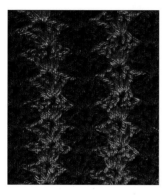

STITCH GLOSSARY
shell (2 dc, ch 1, 2 dc) in indicated st.
rev sc (reverse single crochet, or crab stitch) Insert hook into indicated sp or st in opposite direction than you normally crochet (right hand crocheters insert hook in next st to the right, left hand crocheters insert hook in next st to the left). Draw up a lp, yo and draw through 2 lps on hook.

NOTES
1) Shawl is reversible, with no right or wrong side.
2) After row 2, rows are worked in pairs, with side one facing for two rows, then side two facing for two rows.
3) Shells are always worked in the row below the row you have just completed. For example, row 4 is worked in the ch-1 sps of row 2, row 7 in row 5, etc.
4) The double crochets must be worked over the ch-3 of the opposite color. Do not push the ch-3 in front of or behind the

work, but cover it. After row 3 is complete, shells are always worked in the same color shells: A in A, B in B.
5) Do *not* fasten off yarn for color changes. Drop the working loop of one color where it ends; it will be where you need it.

SHAWL
FIRST HALF
With A, ch 92.
Row 1 2 dc in 4th ch from hook (sk ch counts as dc), *ch 3, sk 7 ch, shell in next ch; rep from * to last 8 ch, ch 3, sk 7 ch, 3 dc in last ch—11 shells.
Row 2 Ch 1, turn, sc in first dc, ch 1, sk 3 ch on foundation ch, shell in next ch on foundation ch (working over the ch-3 sp from row 1), *ch 3, sk shell and 3 ch on foundation ch, shell in next ch on foundation ch; rep from * to t-ch, ch 1, sc in top of t-ch, drop A—12 shells.
Row 3 (side 1 facing) Turn, join B with sl st in first sc, ch 3 (counts as dc throughout), 2 dc in same sc, *ch 3, sk next shell, shell in next ch-1 sp of row below (working over ch-3 sp throughout); rep from * to last shell, ch 3, sk last shell, 3 dc in last sc, drop B.
Row 4 (side 1 facing) Do not turn, pick up A on opposite side of shawl at beg of prev row, ch 1, sc in top of t-ch, ch 1, shell in ch-1 sp of row below, *ch 3, sk next shell, shell in next ch-1 sp of row below; rep from * to last 3 dc, ch 1, sc in last dc, drop A.

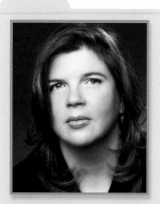

MARY BETH'S STORY
Mary Beth Temple is probably best-known for her podcast *Getting Loopy!*, in which she covers all things crochet and interviews designers and crochet personalities. She's designed and edited patterns for *Vogue Knitting Crochet* and contributed to many other knitting and crochet publications, as well as authoring several books, including *Curvy Girl Crochet*. But crochet isn't her only love; once a Broadway costumer, Mary Beth was able to indulge in her secret talent: singing! She was inspired to contribute to *Crochet Red* after her older sister had a heart attack. Like many women, her sister did not recognize the symptoms and dismissed them at first. Although she sought medical care later than she should have, fortunately she won't suffer long-term effects. However, the episode spurred Mary Beth to get more women thinking about protecting themselves against heart disease. In her own life, she practices yoga to stay fit and manage stress.

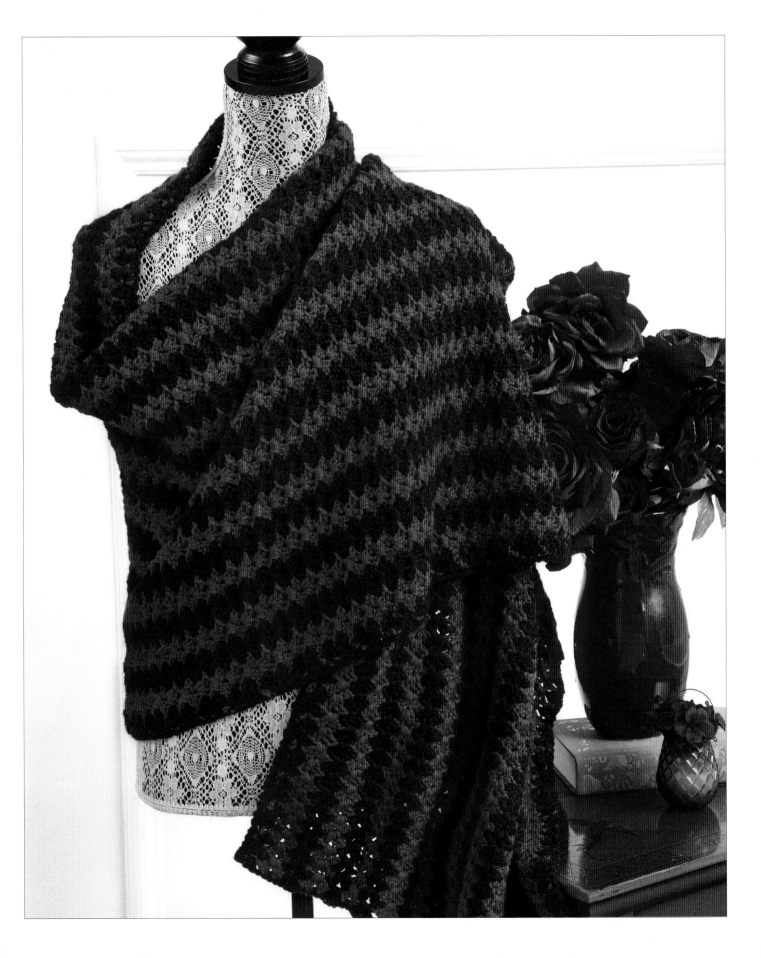

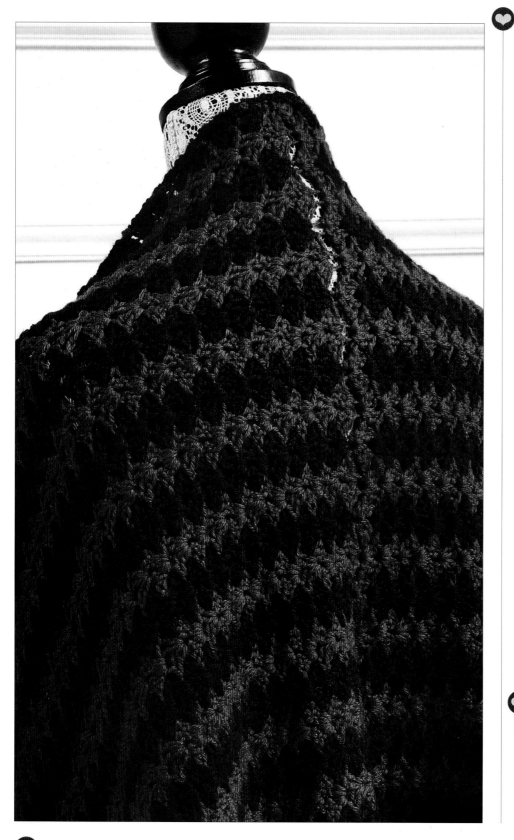

Row 5 (side 2 facing) Turn, pick up B, ch 1, sl st in first sc, ch 3, 2 dc in same sc, *ch 3, sk next shell, shell in next ch-1 sp of row below; rep from * to last shell, ch 3, sk next shell, 3 dc in last sc, drop B.

Row 6 (side 2 facing) Rep row 4. Rep rows 3–6 until piece measures 34½"/87.5cm, ending with an even row in A.

Next row Turn, pick up B, ch 1, sl st in first sc, ch 3, 2 dc in same sc, *ch 1, sc in next (A) shell, ch 1, shell in next ch-1 sp of row below; rep from * to last (A) shell, ch 1, sc in last (A) shell, ch 1, 3 dc in last sc, fasten off.

SECOND HALF

Row 1 Working in opposite side of foundation ch, join A with sc in first foundation ch at base of 3-dc group, ch 1, shell in foundation ch at base of next shell, *ch 3, shell in foundation ch at base of next shell; rep from * to last 4 ch, ch 1, sc in last foundation ch at base of last 3-dc group.
Starting with row 3, work as for first half.

FINISHING

Join yarn to long edge of shawl with sl st.

Row 1 Ch 1, sc evenly across edge, working around row ends.

Row 2 Ch 1, do not turn, rev sc in each sc across, fasten off.
Rep on opposite edge.
Block lightly to measurements. ❤

MARY BETH'S TIP
TAKE UP A HOBBY THAT INVOLVES EXERCISE. Mary Beth supports her daughter's involvement in her own heart-healthy hobby: Irish step dancing!

KRISTIN OMDAHL

Tunisian Shrug

Strips of Tunisian crochet are joined and finished with oversized ribbed cuffs and collar in a garment that makes a dramatic textural statement.

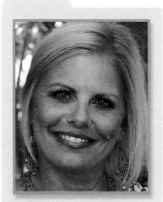

KRISTIN'S STORY
With her innovative techniques and eye for trends, Kristin Omdahl is often credited with bringing crochet back into fashion. When she's not designing, crocheting, or knitting in southwest Florida, you can find Kristin in the "Crochet Corner" of public television's *Knitting Daily*. She has authored several books and is a Craftsy instructor, as well as the brains behind Styled By Kristin, her design company and website. Surprisingly, Kristin took up crochet just eleven years ago, while pregnant. Her geometric, textural designs reflect her love of both math and nature. Heart disease hit home when Kristin's father suffered a heart attack; he has since made a full recovery. A single mom and former model, Kristin knows the importance of keeping in shape and setting a good example. She lifts weights for cardio and strength, and plays football with her son—and last year she began training for a marathon!

SIZES
Instructions are written for size Small/Medium. Changes for sizes Large/X-Large and XX-Large/XXX-Large are in parentheses. (Shown in size Small/Medium.)

MEASUREMENTS
WIDTH (NOT INCLUDING COLLAR AND CUFFS)
30 (30, 35)"/76 (76, 89)cm
LENGTH 16"/40.5cm
WIDTH FROM CUFF TO CUFF
38 (40, 43)"/96.5 (101.5, 109)cm
FRONT OPENING CIRCUMFERENCE
40 (48, 56)"/101.5 (122, 142)cm

MATERIALS
• 6 (6, 6) 3½oz/100g hanks (each approx 140yd/128m) of Skacel Collection *HiKoo SimpliWorsted* (superwash merino/acrylic/nylon) in #046 crimson ④
• Size L/11 (8mm) crochet hook *or size to obtain gauge*
• Tapestry needle

GAUGES
11 sts and 6 rows = 4"/10cm over Tunisian double crochet (Tdc) using size L/11 (8mm) crochet hook.
One strip = 5 x 16"/12.5 x 40.5cm.
➤ Take time to check gauges.

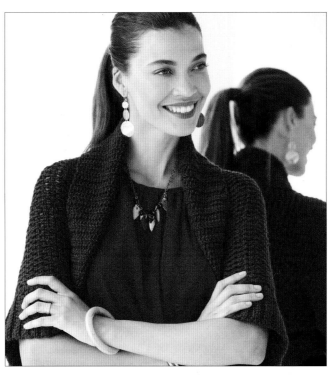

NOTES
1) Shrug is made from 6 (6, 7) Tunisian strips. The strips are joined together as you crochet to form a rectangle. The rectangle is folded and seamed to form front and sleeve openings, then collar and cuffs are worked around the openings.
2) Because only a small number of loops are held on the hook at one time, a Tunisian crochet hook or standard crochet hook with an inline shaft can be used to work the Tunisian strips. The cuffs and collar are worked in standard crochet.

SHRUG
FIRST STRIP
Ch 15.
Row 1 (forward pass) Yo, insert hook in 3rd ch from hook and pull up a lp (3 lps on hook), yo and draw through 2 lps on hook (2 lps remain on hook), *yo, insert hook in next ch and pull up a lp, yo and draw through 2 lps on hook (1 more lp on hook); rep from * across—14 lps on hook.

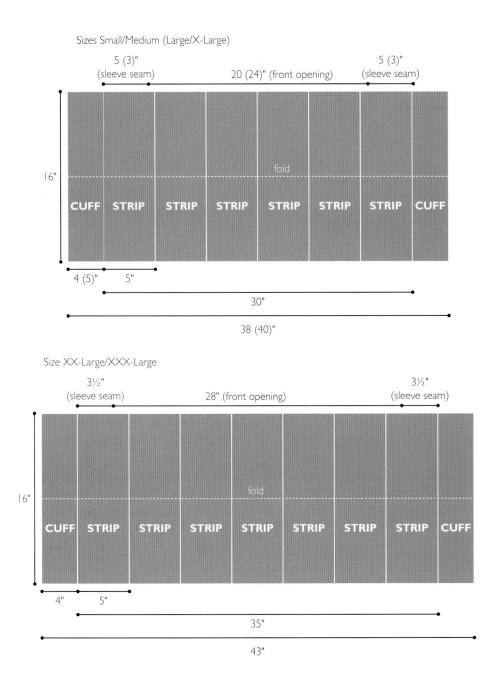

Sizes Small/Medium (Large/X-Large)

5 (3)"
(sleeve seam)

20 (24)" (front opening)

5 (3)"
(sleeve seam)

16"

fold

CUFF STRIP STRIP STRIP STRIP STRIP STRIP CUFF

4 (5)" 5"

30"

38 (40)"

Size XX-Large/XXX-Large

3½"
(sleeve seam)

28" (front opening)

3½"
(sleeve seam)

16"

fold

CUFF STRIP STRIP STRIP STRIP STRIP STRIP STRIP CUFF

4" 5"

35"

43"

Row 1 (return pass) Yo and draw through 1 lp on hook, *yo and draw through 2 lps on hook; rep from * across (1 lp remains on hook)—14 Tunisian double crochet (Tdc).

Row 2 (forward pass) Ch 2 (counts as first Tdc), sk first vertical bar, *yo, insert hook under next vertical bar and pull

up a lp, yo and draw through 2 lps on hook; rep from * across—14 lps on hook.

Row 2 (return pass) Work as for row 1 (return pass)—14 Tdc.

Rows 3–24 Rep last row (forward and return passes) 22 times more.

Row 25 Sl st loosely in each vertical bar across. Fasten off.

SECOND STRIP

Draw up a lp in 14th ch of beg ch of previous strip (at base of beg edge of first row of previous strip), ch 15.

Row 1 (forward pass) Work as for row 1 (forward pass) of first strip—14 lps on hook.

Row 1 (return pass) Insert hook in end of first return row of

previous strip and pull up a lp (15 lps on hook), *yo and draw through 2 lps on hook; rep from * across (1 lp remains on hook)—14 Tdc.

Row 2 (forward pass) Work as for row 2 (forward pass) of first strip—14 lps on hook.

Row 2 (return pass) Insert hook in end of next return row of previous strip and pull up a lp (15 lps on hook), *yo and draw through 2 lps on hook; rep from * across (1 lp remains on hook)—14 Tdc.

Rows 3–24 Rep last row (forward and return passes) 22 times more.

Row 25 Sl st loosely in each vertical bar across. Fasten off.

NEXT 4 (4, 5) STRIPS

Work same as second strip, joining each strip to previous strip. Rectangle now measures approx 30 (30, 35)"/76 (76, 89)cm × 16"/40.5cm. Fold rectangle in half lengthwise, with RS together. Beg at one corner, sew or sl st long edges together for 5 (3, 3½)"/12.5 (7.5, 9)cm to form sleeve. Rep beg at opposite corner. Leave approx 20 (24, 28)"/51 (61, 71)cm unsewn at center for front opening, adjust length of sleeve seams for best fit. Turn piece RS out.

COLLAR

Set-up rnd (RS) With RS facing, join yarn with sl st anywhere in edge of front opening, ch 1, sc evenly spaced all the way around (working 1 sc in each st); join with sl st in first sc.

Note The collar ribbing is now worked back and forth in rows at a right angle to the front opening.

Row 1 Ch 27, hdc in 2nd ch from hook and in each ch across, sl st in next 2 sc of rnd 1—26 hdc and 2 sl sts.

Row 2 Turn, sk the 2 sl sts just made, working in back lps (BL) of sts in previous row, hdc BL in each hdc across—26 hdc.

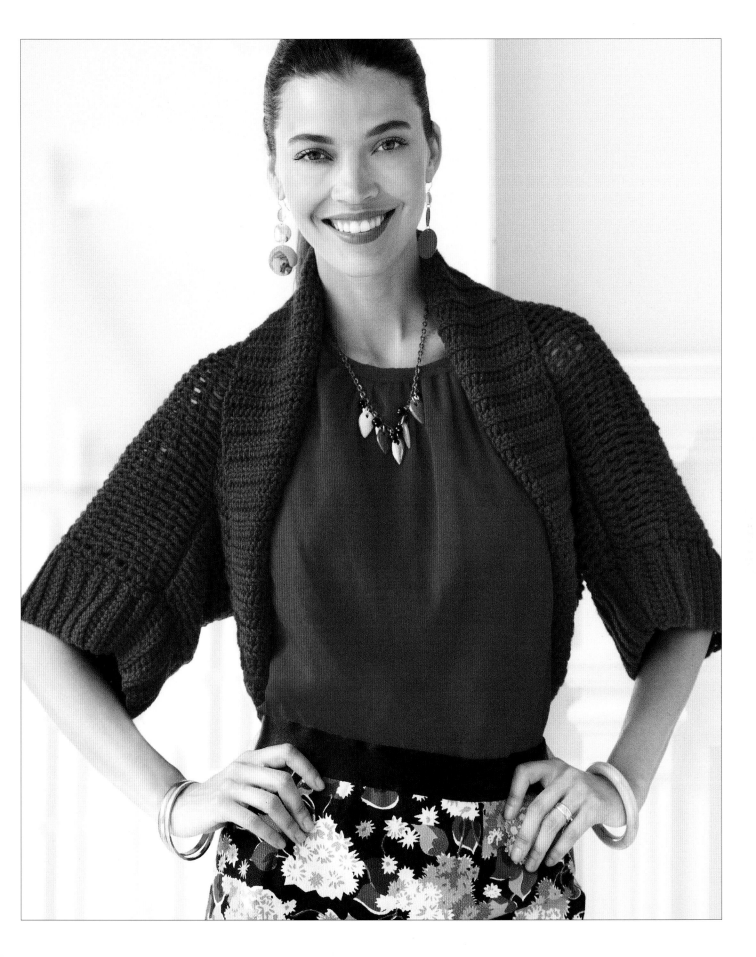

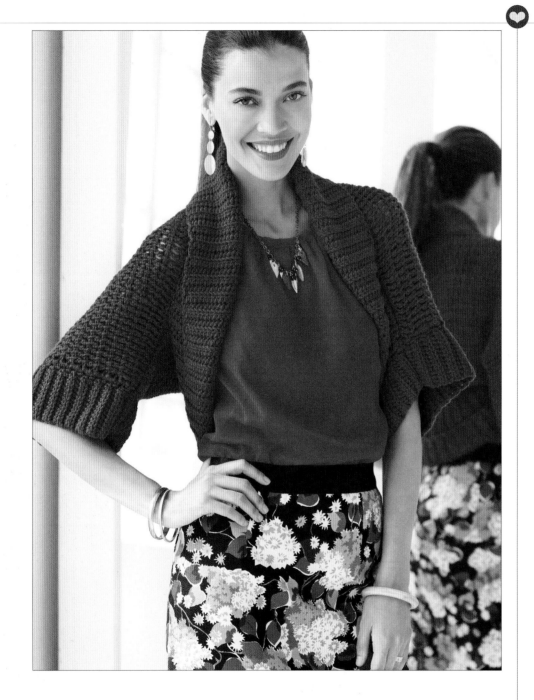

Row 3 Ch 2 (counts as first hdc), turn, hdc BL in each st across, sl st in next 2 sc of rnd 1.
Row 4 Rep row 2.
Rep last 2 rows until you have worked all the way around the front opening. Fasten off, leaving a long tail. With tail, sew or sl st first and last row together.

CUFFS
Set-up rnd (RS) With RS facing, join yarn with sl st anywhere in edge of sleeve opening, ch 1, sc evenly spaced all the way around (working 1 sc in each st); join with sl st in first sc.
Row 1 Ch 13 (16, 13), hdc in 2nd ch from hook and in each ch across, sl st in next 2 sc of rnd 1—12 (15, 12) hdc and 2 sl sts.
Row 2 Turn, sk the 2 sl sts just made, working in back lps (BL) of sts in previous row, hdc BL in each hdc across—12 (15, 12) hdc.
Row 3 Ch 2 (counts as first hdc), turn, hdc BL in each st across, sl st in next 2 sc of rnd 1.
Row 4 Rep row 2.
Rep last 2 rows until you have worked all the way around the sleeve opening. Fasten off, leaving a long tail. With tail, sew or sl st first and last rows together. Rep around other sleeve opening.

FINISHING
Block lightly to measurements. ❤

❤KRISTIN'S TIP
LEAN TOWARD SMALL, HEALTHY MEALS throughout the day and choose lower-carb foods with a good balance of protein and fiber for satiety.

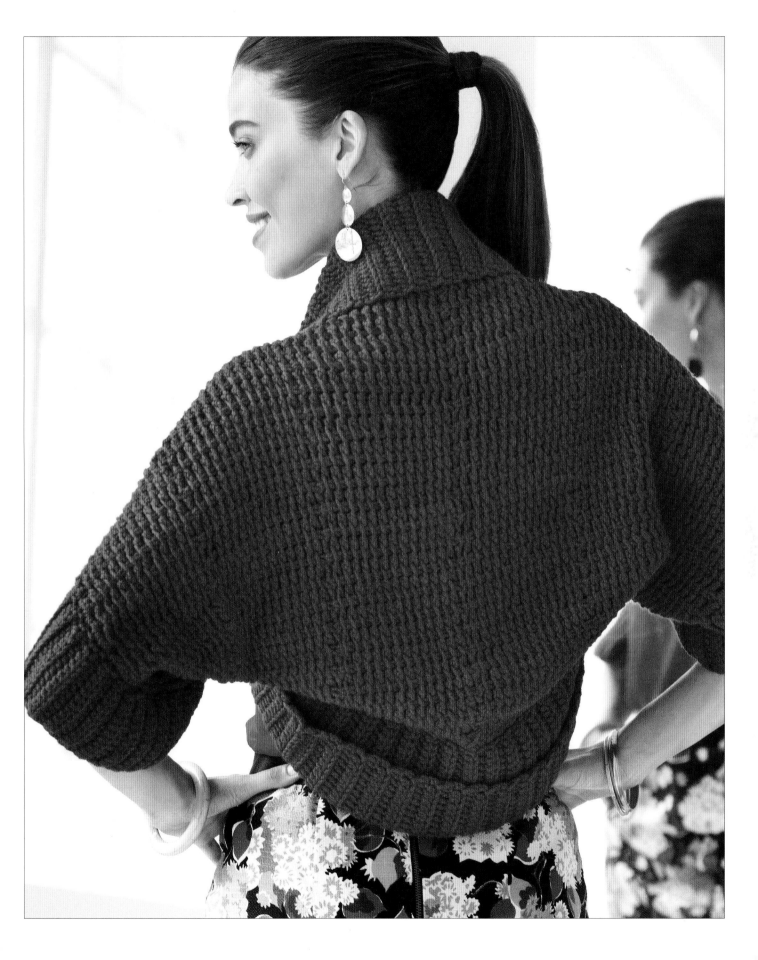

Mitered Brick Throw

A repeating pattern of mitered rectangles worked in a modular construction is both modern and rustic, and a scalloped edging sets it off beautifully.

MEASUREMENTS
WIDTH 43"/109cm
LENGTH 55"/139.5cm

MATERIALS
• 3 3½oz/100g skeins
(each approx 170yd/156m)
of Lion Brand Yarns
Vanna's Choice (acrylic) in
#148 burgundy (A)
• 5 skeins in #180 cranberry (B)
• 2 skeins each in #133 brick
(C) and #113 scarlet (D) (④)
• Size J/10 (8mm) crochet hook
or size to obtain gauge
• Tapestry needle

GAUGE
12 sc and 12 rows = 4"/10cm
over sc using size J/10 (8mm)
crochet hook.
➤Take time to check gauge.

STITCH GLOSSARY
sc3tog (single crochet 3 together)
Insert hook into st and draw up a
lp, [insert hook into next st and
draw up a lp] 2 times, yo, draw
through all 4 lps on hook—2 sts
decreased.

NOTES
1) Afghan is worked in a modular
fashion, working new motifs by
picking up sts along edges of
previous motifs.
Each motif is worked with the
same number of sts. Motif is
worked from outside edges,
decreasing until no sts remain.
Last row and edges of rows
create a long straight top edge
with first row creating remaining
3 outside edges of motif. Next
motif is worked along one short
edge of previous motif, adding
new sts until same number of sts
and is worked in same manner as
first motif. New motifs are added
until first row of motifs has been
joined. Second row of motifs is
worked along edges of first row.
Motifs are joined in rows,
beginning at lower right corner
and ending at upper left corner.
2) When changing colors, work
last step of last st of previous
color with new color.

THROW
FIRST MOTIF
With A, ch 55.
Row 1 Sc in 2nd ch from hook, sc
in next 11 ch, sc3tog, sc in next
24 ch, sc3tog, sc in next 12 ch,
turn—50 sts.

Row 2 Ch 1, sc in next 11 sc,
sc3tog, sc in next 22 sc, sc3tog, sc
in next 11 sc, change to B in last
st, turn—46 sts.
Row 3 Ch 1, sc in next 10 sc,
sc3tog, sc in next 20 sc, sc3tog, sc
in next 10 sc, turn—42 sts.
Row 4 Ch 1, sc in next 9 sc,
sc3tog, sc in next 18 sc, sc3tog, sc
in next 9 sc, turn—38 sts.
Row 5 Ch 1, sc in next 8 sc,
sc3tog, sc in next 16 sc, sc3tog, sc
in next 8 sc, turn—34 sts.
Row 6 Ch 1, sc in next 7 sc,
sc3tog, sc in next 14 sc, sc3tog, sc
in next 7 sc, change to C in last st,
turn—30 sts.
Row 7 Ch 1, sc in next 6 sc,
sc3tog, sc in next 12 sc, sc3tog, sc
in next 6 sc, turn—26 sts.
Row 8 Ch 1, sc in next 5 sc,
sc3tog, sc in next 10 sc, sc3tog, sc
in next 5 sc, change to D in last
st, turn—22 sts.
Row 9 Ch 1, sc in next 4 sc,
sc3tog, sc in next 8 sc, sc3tog, sc
in next 4 sc, turn—18 sts.
Row 10 Ch 1, sc in next 3 sc,
sc3tog, sc in next 6 sc, sc3tog, sc
in next 3 sc, turn—14 sts.
Row 11 Ch 1, sc in next 2 sc,
sc3tog, sc in next 4 sc, sc3tog, sc
in next 2 sc, turn—10 sts.
Row 12 Ch 1, sc in next sc,
sc3tog, sc in next 2 sc, sc3tog, sc
in next sc, turn—6 sts.
Row 13 Ch 1, skip first sc, sc in
next 2 sc, sl st in last st, fasten off.

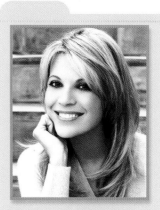

VANNA'S STORY
Between her thirty-year run
on *Wheel of Fortune* and her
appearances in movies and on
TV, Vanna White is one of the
most recognizable figures in
American pop culture. She's
also a mother, a crafter and
designer, and the creator of a
popular line of yarn with Lion
Brand. Her grandmother
taught her to crochet when
she was a girl, and she's
passed on the craft to her two
daughters. Vanna once wanted
to be a nurse; caring for
others comes naturally to her,
and half the proceeds from
her yarn sales go to St. Jude
Children's Research Hospital.
Raising awareness about heart
disease is a family tradition:
Vanna's mother volunteered
yearly at the Myrtle Beach
telethon to raise money for
the cause. Vanna cares for her
health with regular exercise—
she spins on a stationary bike
daily—and with another
healthy habit that's often
overlooked: getting plenty
of sleep!

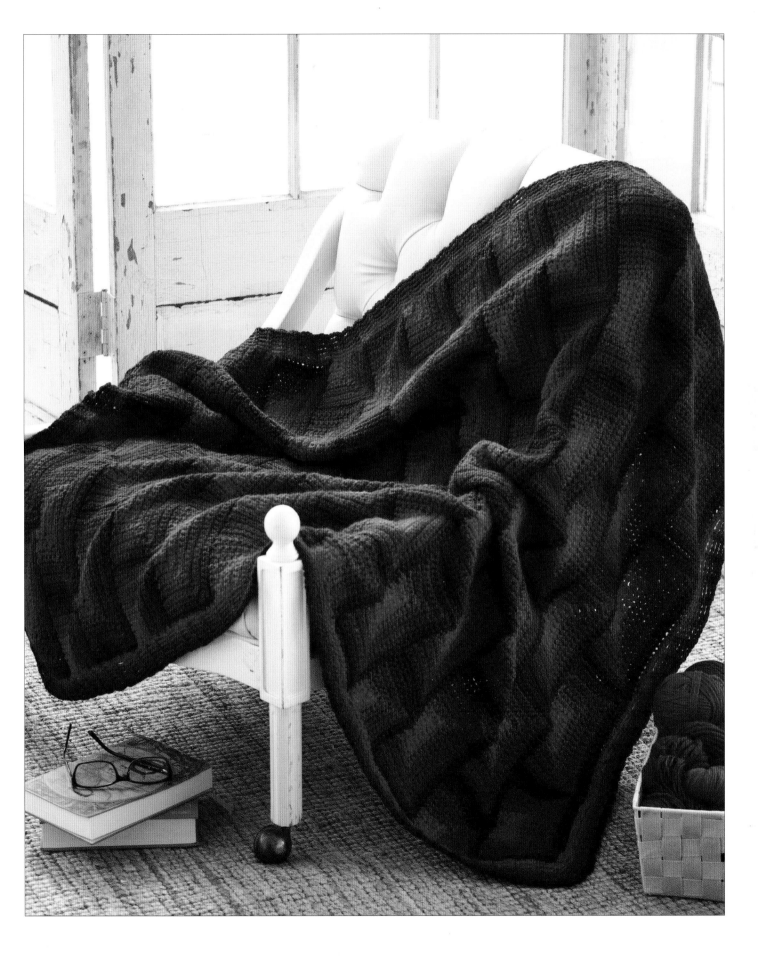

SECOND MOTIF

Holding first motif with first row as side and lower edges and last row and row edges as long straight top edge, join A at lower left corner of first motif, ch 42.

Row 1 Sc in 2nd ch from hook, sc in next 11 ch, sc3tog, sc in next 24 ch, sc3tog, sc 12 sts evenly spaced along short edge of previous motif—50 sts.
Work rows 2–13 as for first motif.

THIRD, FOURTH, AND FIFTH MOTIFS

Work as for second motif, adding motifs in a row from right to left.

SECOND ROW
FIRST HALF MOTIF

Working from right to left, join A at center point of first motif of first row, ch 14.

Row 1 Sc in 2nd ch from hook, sc in next 11 ch, sc3tog, sc 12 sts evenly spaced along first half of first motif, turn—25 sts.

Row 2 Ch 1, sc in next 11 sc, sc3tog, sc in next 11 sc, change to B in last st, turn—23 sts.

Row 3 Ch 1, turn, sc in next 10 sc, sc3tog, sc in next 10 sc, turn—21 sts.

Row 4 Ch 1, sc in next 9 sc, sc3tog, sc in next 9 s, turn—19 sts.

Row 5 Ch 1, sc in next 8 sc, sc3tog, sc in next 8 sc, turn—17 sts.

Row 6 Ch 1, sc in next 7 sc, sc3tog, sc in next 7 sc, change to C in last st, turn—15 sts.

Row 7 Ch 1, sc in next 6 sc, sc3tog, sc in next 6 sc—13 sts.

Row 8 Ch 1, sc in next 5 sc, sc3tog, sc in next 5 sc, change to D in last st, turn—11 sts.

Row 9 Ch 1, sc in next 4 sc, sc3tog, sc in next 4 sc, turn—9 sts.

Row 10 Ch 1, sc in next 3 sc, sc3tog, sc in next 3 sc, turn—7 sts.

Row 11 Ch 1, sc in next 2 sc, sc3tog, sc in next 2 sc, turn—5 sts.

Row 12 Ch 1, sc in next sc, sc3tog, sc in next sc, turn—3 sts.

Row 13 Ch 1, skip first sc, sc in next sc, sl st in last st, fasten off.

SECOND, THIRD, AND FOURTH MOTIFS

Working from right to left, join A at center of next motif, ch 14.

Row 1 Sc in 2nd ch from hook, sc in next 11 ch, sc3tog, sc 24 sts evenly spaced from center of motif to center of previous motif, sc3tog, sc 12 sts evenly spaced along short edge of previous motif—50 sts.
Work rows 2–13 as for first motif.

LAST HALF MOTIF

Row 1 Join A at first row of last motif on previous row, ch 1, sc 12 sts evenly spaced to center of last motif, sc3tog, 12 sc evenly spaced along short edge of previous motif—25 sts.
Work rows 2–13 as for first half motif.

THIRD ROW
FIRST MOTIF

Join A at last st of first half motif of previous row, ch 14 and fasten off.
Join A at center of next motif, ch 14.

Row 1 Sc in 2nd ch from hook, sc in next 11 ch, sc3tog, sc 24 sts evenly spaced along edge to 1 st before first 14-ch just made, sc3tog, sc in next 12 ch, turn—50 sts. Work as for first motif.

SECOND–FIFTH MOTIFS

Working from right to left, join A at center of next motif, ch 14.

Row 1 Sc in 2nd ch from hook, sc in next 11 ch, sc3tog, sc 24 sts evenly spaced from center of motif to center of previous motif, sc3tog, sc 12 sts evenly spaced along short edge of previous motif—50 sts.
Work rows 2–13 as for first motif. Alternate 2nd and 3rd rows until there are 13 motif rows.

FINISHING
EDGING

Rnd 1 Join D in any corner, ch 1, *sc in corner, sc 131 sts evenly spaced along short edge, sc in corner, sc 171 sts evenly spaced along long edge; rep from * once more, slip st in first st—608 sc.

Rnd 2 Ch 1, sc in corner st, *(ch 2, sc) in same corner st, [ch 3, skip 3 sts, sc in next sc] to corner st; rep from * around, ch 2, slip st in first sc. Fasten off.

Rnd 3 Join C and rep rnd 2, working 3 ch at each corner. Fasten off.

Rnd 4 Join B and rep rnd 2, working 5 ch at each corner. Fasten off.

Rnd 5 Join A and rep rnd 2, working 7 ch at each corner. Fasten off.❤

❤ VANNA'S TIP

VANNA MADE IT HER NEW YEAR'S RESOLUTION to try out a new healthy recipe each week. What a great way to make healthy food and keep it interesting at the same time!

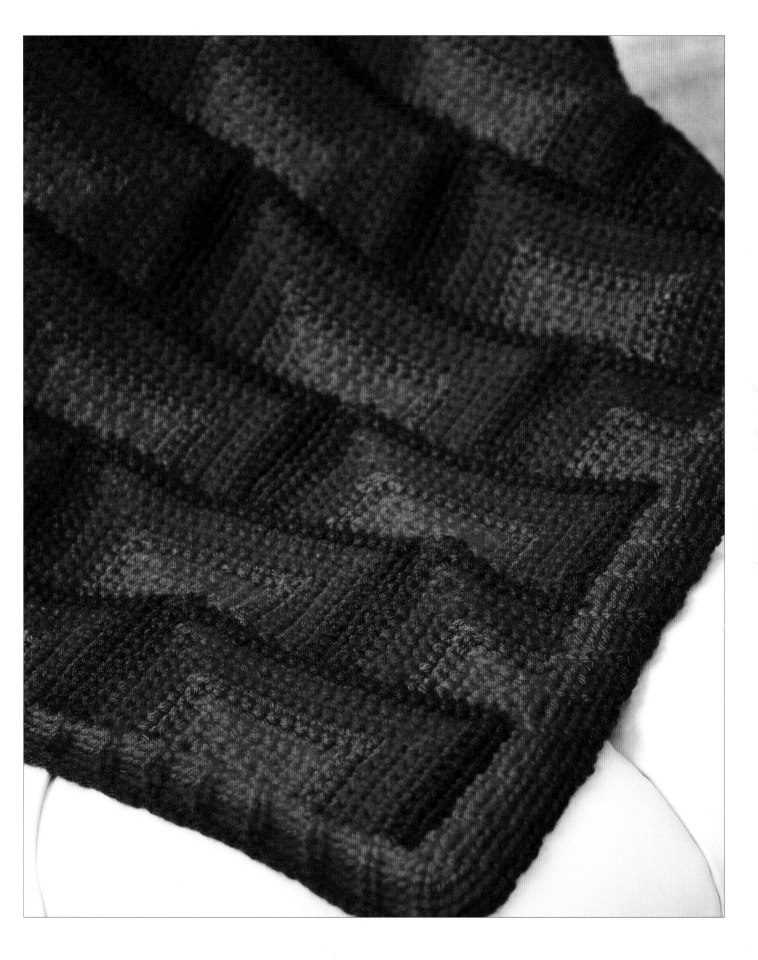

Vortex Slouchy Hat

A super-slouchy hat gets an extra dose of style from a swirling pattern of clusters and eyelets that comes together at the crown.

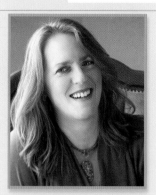

SIZES
Instructions are written for size Small. Changes for Medium and Large are in parentheses. (Shown in size Small.)

MEASUREMENTS
BRIM CIRCUMFERENCE
18 (20½, 23)"/45.5 (52, 58.5)cm
HEIGHT
11 (11½, 12)"/28 (29, 30.5)cm

MATERIALS
• 2 (2, 2) 1¾oz/50g hanks (each approx 146yd/135m) of Tahki Yarns/Tahki • Stacy Charles *Cotton Classic Lite* (mercerized cotton) in #4997 bright red (❷)
• Size F/5 (3.75mm) crochet hook *or size to obtain gauge*
• Tapestry needle

GAUGE
8 rnds = 6½"/16.5cm over pat st using size F/5 (3.75mm) crochet hook.
➤ Take time to check gauge.

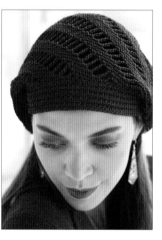

STITCH GLOSSARY
beg Cl (beginning cluster) Ch 4, *yo twice, insert hook in indicated space and draw up a lp, [yo and draw through 2 lps on hook] twice; rep from * once more in *same* space, yo and draw through all 3 lps on hook.
3tr-Cl (3 treble crochet cluster) *Yo twice, insert hook in indicated space and draw up a lp, [yo and draw through 2 lps on hook] twice; rep from * twice more in *same* space, yo and draw through all 4 lps on hook.

NOTE
Hat is worked on the right side only without turning throughout.

HAT
Ch 8, join with sl st in first ch to form a ring.
Rnd 1 (RS) Ch 5 (counts as dc and ch-2 sp), *dc in ring, ch 2; rep from * 10 times more, join with sl st to 3rd ch of beg ch—12 dc.

Rnd 2 Beg Cl in ch-sp made by beg ch, *ch 4, 3tr-Cl in next ch-2 sp; rep from * around, ch 1, join with dc in top of beg Cl.
Rnd 3 Ch 1, sc around post of dc, ch 5, *sc in next ch-4 sp, ch 5; rep from * around, join with sl st in first sc.
Rnd 4 Ch 1, sc in first sc, 2 sc in next ch-5 sp, ch 5, *sc in next sc, 2 sc in next ch-5 sp, ch 5; rep from * around, join with sl st in first sc.
Rnd 5 Ch 1, *sk 1 sc, sc in next 2 sc, 2 sc in next ch-5 sp, ch 5; rep from * around, join with sl st in first sc.
Rnd 6 Ch 1, *sk 1 sc, sc in next 3 sc, 2 sc in next ch-5 sp, ch 5; rep from * around, join with sl st in first sc.
Rnd 7 Ch 1, *sk 1 sc, sc in next 4 sc, 2 sc in next ch-5 sp, ch 5; rep from * around, join with sl st in first sc.
Rnd 8 Ch 1, *sk 1 sc, sc in next 5 sc, 2 sc in next ch-5 sp, ch 5; rep from * around, join with sl st in first sc.
Rnd 9 Ch 1, *sk 1 sc, sc2tog over next 2 sc, sc in each of next 4 sc, 2 sc in next ch-5 sp, ch 5; rep from * around, join with sl st in first sc.
Rep rnd 9 until hat measures 9 (9¼, 9½)"/23 (23.5, 24)cm from center of crown.

JILL'S STORY
A native of England, Jill Wright learned to crochet from a neighbor when she was eight and hasn't put down her hook since. She also learned to knit and sew from her mother—the start of a lifelong love affair with the fiber arts. She made baby clothes to earn Girl Scout badges and finished her first full-size garment at age fourteen! Jill enjoys many other crafts as well: beading, macramé, spinning, felting, and drawing, to name a few. She turned her crafting into a career so she could stay home with her sons. Heart disease and related problems run in Jill's family: her grandmother had high blood pressure, and her aunt died of a heart attack. Her family history, combined with her own struggles with high cholesterol, inspired Jill to take steps to improve her personal health—including long walks with her dog, Wiggie.

♥ **JILL'S TIP**
JILL STARTS EACH DAY WITH A BOWL OF OATMEAL topped with almonds, raspberries, and flax seeds—a high-fiber, lowfat breakfast that gives her tons of energy and plenty of antioxidants.

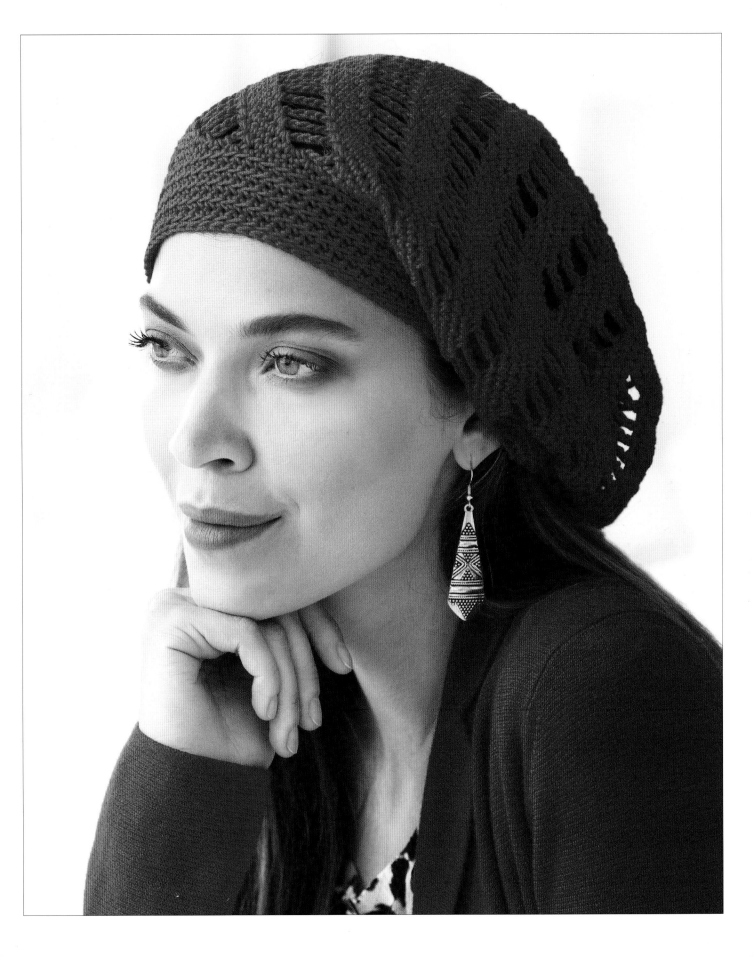

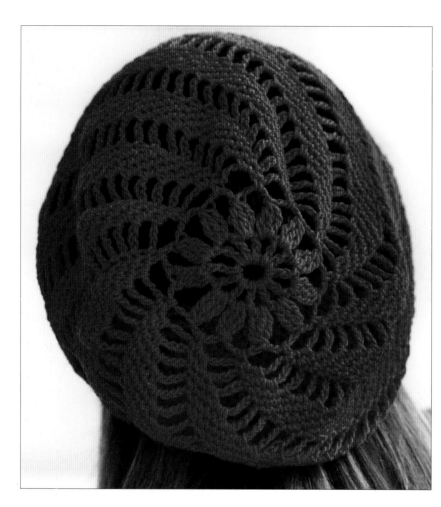

SHAPING
Rnd 1 Ch 1, *sk 1 sc, sc2tog over next 2 sc, sc in each of next 4 sc, 2 sc in next 5 ch-sp, ch 3 (3, 4); rep from * around, join with sl st in first sc.
Rnd 2 Ch 1, *sk 1 sc, sc2tog over next 2 sc, sc in each of next 4 sc, 2 sc in next ch-sp, ch 1 (2, 3); rep from * around, join with sl st in first sc.
Rnd 3 Ch 1, *sc in each of next 6 sc, 1 (2, 3) sc in next ch-sp; rep from * around, sl st in first sc—84 (96, 108) sc.

BAND
Rnd 1 Ch 1, sc tbl in each sc around, join with sl st to first sc.
Rnd 2 Ch 1, sc tfl in each sc around, join with sl st to first sc.
Rep rnds 1 and 2 until band measures 1½ (1¾, 2)"/4 (4.5, 5)cm, fasten off.

FINISHING
Block lightly to measurements. ❤

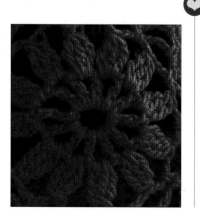

STITCH KEY
- •   sl st
- ⬭   ch
- ┼   sc
- ┬   dc
- ⬙   CL3
- ⋏   sc2tog

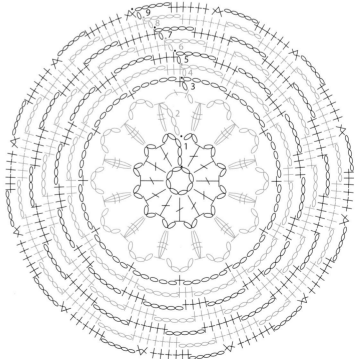

VICKIE HOWELL

Yoga Bag

A simple, open mesh pattern and a fabric-lined handle make a caddy for your yoga mat that will get you to the gym in style.

■■□□

MEASUREMENTS
LENGTH
26"/66cm
CIRCUMFERENCE
16"/40.5cm

MATERIALS
• 1 2.4oz/70g skein (each approx 282yd/258m) of Bernat *Cotton-ish by Vickie Howell* (cotton/acrylic) in #85434 crimson twine **3**
• Size G/6 (4mm) crochet hook *or size to obtain gauge*
• Tapestry needle
• 28½"/72.5cm × 1½"/4cm piece of cotton fabric
• Coordinating thread and sewing needle

GAUGE
14 sts/2 pat reps and 4 rows = 3½"/9cm over shell pat using size G/6 (4mm) crochet hook.
➤Take time to check gauge.

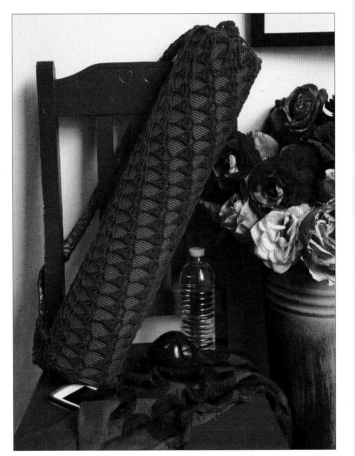

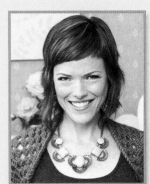

VICKIE'S STORY
Vickie Howell does it all: she designs, writes, hosts, and consults for HGTV's *Knitty Gritty*, is a spokeswoman for Craft Corps, which encourages crafters to share their stories, and is also a busy mom! So we're overjoyed that she contributed a design to *Crochet Red*. Vickie supports other great causes: she founded the Purple Stitch Project to help children with seizure disorders, and is active in the Epilepsy Foundation. Vickie lives in trendy, artistic Austin, where she finds inspiration in the people and sights, including vintage shops—anything bright is liable to catch her eye! Vickie's family is fortunate enough to have avoided heart disease, but she's still aware of the risk: Texas was named in a study of areas prone to obesity, a huge indicator for heart problems. Luckily, she's a fantastic and healthy cook: her vegetarian chili could win a chili cook-off, even in Texas!

STITCH GLOSSARY
Hdc2tog Yo, insert hook in indicated st and draw up a lp, yo, insert hook in next st and draw up a lp, yo, draw through all 5 lps on hook.
FPhdc Yo, insert hook around post of next st at front of work, inserting hook from right to left, yo, pull through post, yo, draw through all lps on hook.

BPhdc Yo, insert hook around post of next st at front of work, inserting hook from left to right, yo, pull through post, yo, draw through all lps on hook.

NOTES
1) Bag is worked from the top down in the round. Do not turn work at the end of each rnd.

BAG

Ch 66, sl st in first ch to form ring, being careful not to twist.

Rnd 1 Ch 2 (counts as 1 hdc here and throughout), hdc in next ch and in each ch around. Join rnd with sl st in top of beg-ch, do not turn—66 sts.

Rnd 2 Ch 2, hdc in each hdc around. Join rnd with sl st in top of beg-ch.

Rnd 3 Ch 3 (counts as 1 hdc and ch-1 here only), *sk 1 hdc, hdc in next hdc, ch 1; rep from * around. Join rnd with sl st in top of beg-ch—33 ch-1 sps.

Rnd 4 Ch 2, hdc in each hdc and ch-1 sp around, working 3 decreases (hdc2tog) evenly spaced around. Join rnd with sl st in top of beg-ch—63 hdc.

Rnd 5 Ch 4 (counts as 1 tr here and throughout), 2 tr in same st as ch, sk 2 hdc, dc in next hdc, *ch 3, sk 3 hdc, 3 tr in next hdc, sk 2 hdc, dc in next hdc; rep from * around, ch 3. Join rnd with sl st at top of beg-ch—9 3-tr shells.

Rnd 6 Sl st in each of next 3 tr and in next dc, ch 4, 2 tr in same dc, dc in next ch-3 sp, *ch 3, sk 3 tr, 3 tr in next dc, dc in next ch-3 sp, rep from * around, ch 3. Join rnd with sl st in top of beg-ch.
Rep rnd 6 until piece measures 26"/66cm from beg edge.

BOTTOM

Rnd 1 Ch 3, work 59 dc evenly spaced around. Join rnd with sl st in top of beg-ch—60 dc counting beg-ch-3.

Rnd 2 Ch 3 (counts as 1 dc), dc in each of next 2 dc, dc2tog, *dc in each of next 3 dc, dc2tog; rep from * around. Join rnd with a sl st in top of beg ch—48 dc.

Rnd 3 Ch 3, dc in next dc, dc2tog, *dc in each of next 2 dc, dc2tog; rep from * around. Join rnd with a sl st in top of beg ch—36 dc.

Rnd 4 Ch 3, dc2tog, *dc in next dc, dc2tog; rep from * around. Join rnd with a sl st in top of beg ch—24 dc.

Rnd 5 Ch 3, hdc in next dc (this counts as 1 dec), dc2tog around. Join rnd with sl st in top of beg-ch—12 dc.

Rnd 6 Rep rnd 5—6 dc. Fasten off, leaving a long tail.

FINISHING

Thread tail into tapestry needle, weave through tops of 6 rem sts and draw tight to close opening.

STRAP
Ch 9.

Row 1 Hdc in 3rd ch from hook and in each ch across—7 hdc.

Row 2 Ch 2, turn, [FPhdc, BPhdc] twice, FPhdc, hdc.

Row 3 Ch 2, turn, (BPhdc, FPhdc) twice, BPhdc, hdc.
Rep rows 2 and 3 until strap measures 28"/71cm. Fasten off.

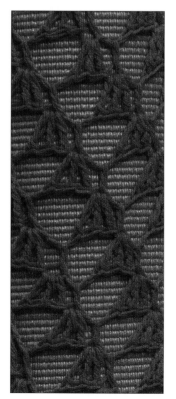

STRAP LINING

With WS facing, press fabric edges in ¼"/.5cm around, so you have a neat strip that's 1"/2.5cm wide. Pin fabric to underside of strap. Hand tack to strap, taking care to ease crocheted fabric as you go along.
Sew strap ends securely to top and bottom of backside of bag.

DRAWSTRING

Crochet a 32"/81cm chain. Fasten off; trim ends.
Feed drawstring through ch-1 sps in rnd 3 and tie.❤

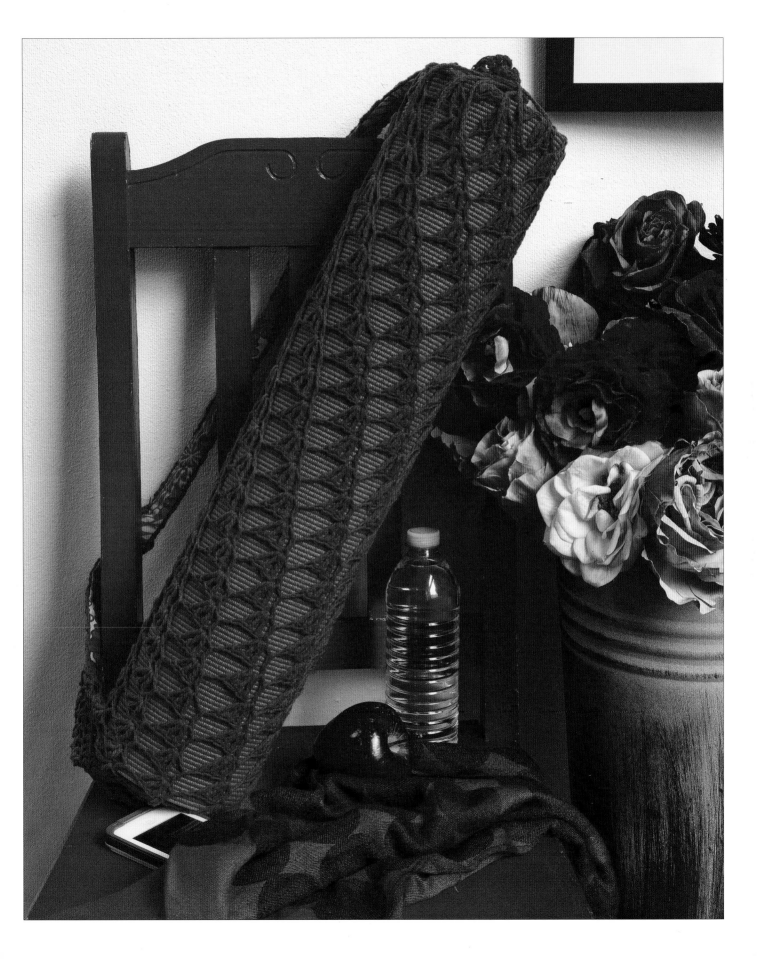

Mock Neck Vest

Paired with a sheath dress or with jeans, this funky long vest with a button collar is a unique scene-stealer. Wear it loose or cinch it with a belt.

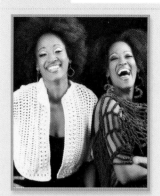

SIZES
Instructions are written for size Small/Medium. Changes for Large and X-Large are in parentheses. (Shown in size Small/Medium.)

MEASUREMENTS
BUST
35½ (44 ½)"/90 (113)cm
LENGTH
28¾ (32¾)"/73 (83)cm

MATERIALS
• 2 5oz/141g skeins (each approx 256yd/234m) of Red Heart *Soft Yarn* (acrylic) in #9925 really red (A)
• 2 skeins in #5142 cherry red (B)
• Size I/9 (5.5mm) crochet hook *or size to obtain gauge*
• Removable stitch markers
• 1 button, 1"/2.5cm diameter

GAUGE
14 dc and 8 rows = 4"/10cm over dc using size I/9 (5.5mm) crochet hook.
➤ Take time to check gauge.

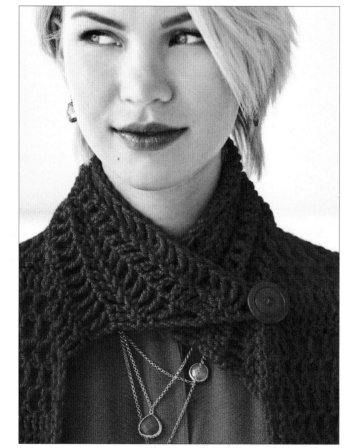

RIGHT FRONT PANEL
Using A, ch 51 (63).
Row 1 Sk 3 ch (counts as 1 dc), dc in 4th ch from hook and in each ch to end—49 (61) dc.
Row 2 Ch 3 (counts as 1 dc here and throughout), dc in next dc, *ch 1, sk next dc, dc in next dc; rep from * to last dc, dc in last dc—23 (29) ch-1 sps.
Rows 3 and 5 Ch 3, dc in next dc, dc in next ch-1 sp, *ch 1, sk next dc, dc in next ch-1 sp; rep from * to last 2 dc, dc in each of last 2 dc—22 (28) ch-1 sps.
Rows 4 and 6 Ch 3, dc in next dc, *ch 1, sk next dc, dc in next ch-1 sp; rep from * to last 3 dc, ch 1, sk next dc, dc in each of last 2 dc—23 (29) ch-1 sps.

SIZE LARGE/X-LARGE ONLY
Row 7 Rep row 5.

ERIKA AND MONIKA'S STORY
Chicago natives Erika and Monika Simmons, aka the Double Stitch Twins, learned to crochet at age ten and knew it was the craft for them. This dream team catapulted into the fashion world as designers, models, and creators of the popular Crochet Fashionista Workshop. The twins have a partnership with the original Macy's in Chicago and are spokespersons and designers for Red Heart yarn. They've even broken into the celebrity world, catching the eye of stars such as Eve and Jennifer Hudson with their fresh designs! Tragedy hit close to home in 2012, when their cousin Davida passed away from a stroke. At forty-one, she was only one year older than the twins—a powerful reminder to care for their health. Happily, they're doing great: Monika practices interval training and chases after her four-year-old daughter, while Erika loves going to Zumba classes.

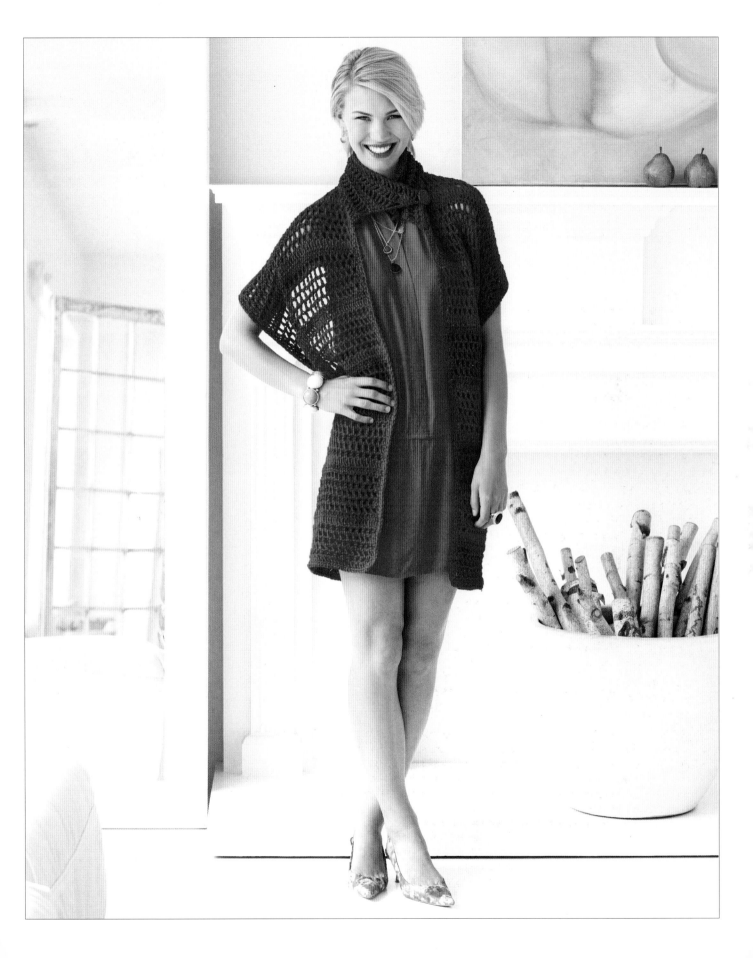

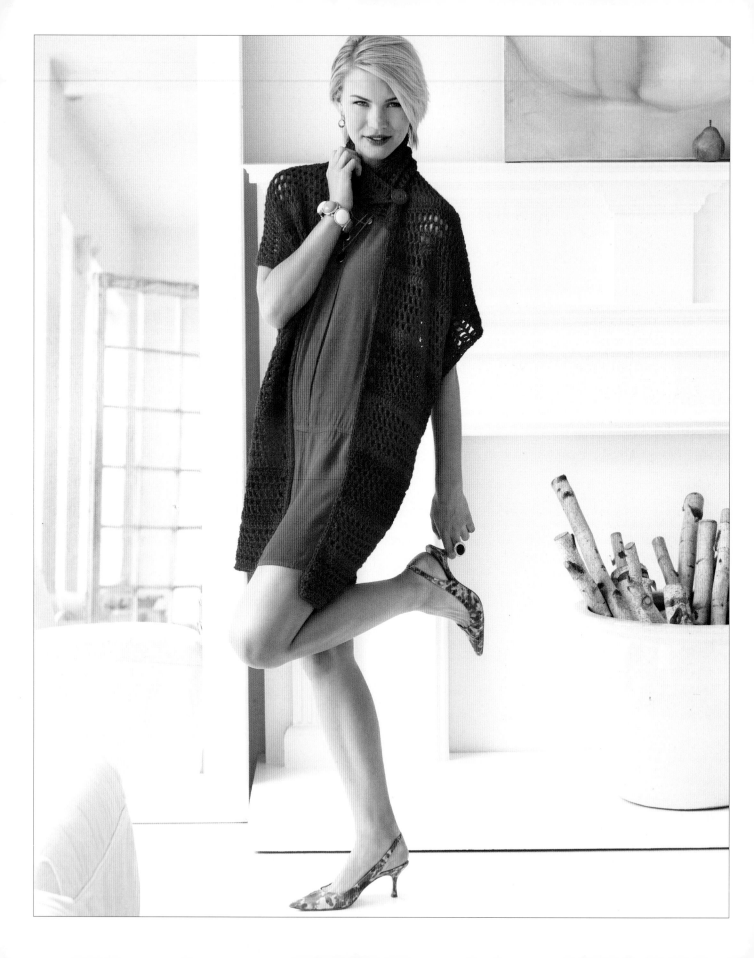

BOTH SIZES

Row 7 (8) Ch 3, dc in each dc and ch-1 sp across—49 (61) dc. Change to B.
Row 8 (9) Ch 3, dc in each dc across—49 (61) dc.
Rows 9–14 (10–16) Rep rows 2–7.
*Change to A and rep rows 8–14 (9–16), change to B and rep rows 8–14 (9–16); rep from * twice more. Do not fasten off.

TRIM

Rotate piece 90 degrees, ch 2, work 92 (104) hdc evenly down long side edge, ch 2, hdc in each st across foundation, ch 2, work 92 (104) hdc evenly down other long side edge, ch 2, hdc in each st across top edge, ch 2, join with sl st in beg ch-2. Fasten off.

LEFT FRONT PANEL

Work same as right front panel, substituting A for B, and B for A.

RIGHT BACK PANEL

With RS facing, join A at left side edge of right front panel, 50 (62) sts up from bottom edge.
Row 1 (RS) Ch 3, dc in each hdc to end—50 (62) dc.
Rows 2–6 (2–8) Ch 3, dc in each dc across.
Fasten off.

LEFT BACK PANEL

With RS facing, join B at bottom right corner of left front panel.
Row 1 (RS) Ch 3, dc in each of the next 49 (61) dc—50 (62) dc.
Rows 2–6 (2–8) Ch 3, dc in each dc across.
Do not fasten off.

FINISHING

JOIN BACK PANELS

With WS facing, sc across final rows of both pieces at the same time. Fasten off.

JOIN FRONT PANELS

With WS facing and top (short) edges of front panels together, use B to sc across outer 4 (5)"/10 (12.5)cm of final rows of both pieces at the same time. Fasten off.

COLLAR

Place markers at each side of top center 18 (20)"/45.5 (51)cm of vest. With RS facing, join A at first marker.
Row 1 (RS) Ch 4 (counts as 1 tr here and throughout), work 47 (53) more tr evenly spaced to next marker—48 (54) tr.
Rows 2 and 3 Ch 4, tr in each tr across.
Row 4 Ch 8, tr in each tr across.
Rows 5 and 6 Ch 8, tr in each tr across, tr in each of the next 4 ch—52 (58) tr.
Row 7 Ch 8, sl st in next tr—56 (62) tr. Fasten off.
Sew button to WS, 2½"/6.5cm in from left corner of collar base. Button will be visible when collar is worn folded out. ❤

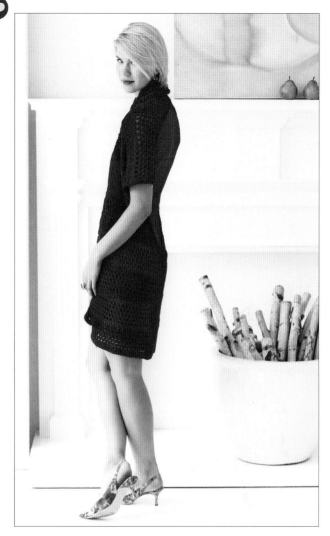

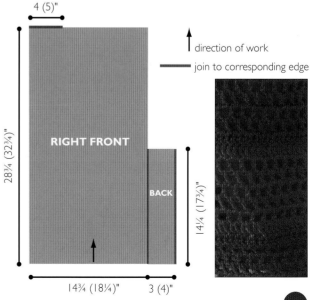

4 (5)"

direction of work

join to corresponding edge

28¾ (32¾)"

RIGHT FRONT

BACK

14¼ (17¾)"

14¾ (18¼)"   3 (4)"

MARLY BIRD

Sweater with Cowl

A perfect layering piece for any season is crocheted in two luxuriously soft yarns, with three-quarter sleeves and an attached cowl.

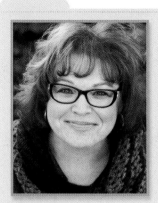

SIZES
Instructions are written for size X-Small. Changes for Small. Medium, Large, and X-Large are in parentheses. (Shown in size Small.)

MEASUREMENTS
BUST
35 (39½, 42, 46½, 51½)"/89 (100, 106.5, 118, 130.5)cm
LENGTH
26 (26, 27, 28, 29½)"/66 (66, 68.5, 71, 75)cm

MATERIALS
• 3 (4, 4, 5, 6) 3½oz/100g hanks (each approx 328yd/300m) of Bijou Spun *Sport Weight* (yak) in deep red (A) (2)
• 3 (3, 4, 4, 4) 1¾oz/50g balls (each approx 435yd/398m) of Bijou Spun *Seraphim* (angora/viscose) in pomegranate (B) (0)
• Size F/5 (3.75mm) crochet hook *or size to obtain gauge*
• Tapestry needle

GAUGE
6 reps and 14 rows = 7"/18cm over asymmetrical pat using size F/5 (3.75 mm) crochet hook.
➤Take time to check gauge.

STITCH GLOSSARY
Dc2tog (double crochet 2 together) Yo and pull up a loop in next dc, yo and draw through 2 loops, sk next dc, yo and pull up a loop in next dc, yo and draw through 2 loops, yo and draw through all 3 loops on hook—2 sts decreased.

ASYMMETRICAL PATTERN
(multiple of 7 sts plus 4)
Row 1 (RS) (4 dc, ch 2, dc) in 7th ch from hook, [sk 6 ch, (4 dc, ch 2, dc) in next ch] to last 4 ch, sk 3 ch, dc in last ch.
Row 2 Ch 2, [(4 dc, ch 2, dc) in next ch-2 sp] across, dc in t-ch. Rep row 2 for asymmetrical pat.

ASYMMETRICAL PATTERN DECREASES
Dec row 1 Ch 4, (dc, ch 2, dc) in 1st ch-2 sp, [(4 dc, ch 2, dc) in next ch-2 sp] to last ch-2 sp, 4 dc in last ch-2 sp, tr in t-ch.
Dec row 2 Ch 3, (dc, ch 1, dc) in 1st dc, [(4 dc, ch 2, dc) in next ch-2 sp] to last ch-2 sp, 3 dc in last ch-2 sp, dc in t-ch.
Dec row 3 Ch 4, [(4 dc, ch 2, dc) in next ch-2 sp] across, sk last ch-1 sp, tr in t-ch.

PINEAPPLE PATTERN
(multiple of 21 sts plus 3)
Row 1 (RS) (Dc, ch 1, dc) in 7th ch from hook, ch 2, sk 4 ch, *(dc, ch 1, dc) in next ch, ch 2, sk 3 ch, (dc, ch 1, dc) in next ch, ch 2, sk 4 ch, (dc, ch 1, dc) in next ch, ch 2, sk 3 ch, (dc, ch 1, dc) in next ch,

ch 2, sk 2 ch, (dc, ch 1, dc) in next ch, ch 2, sk 4 ch, (dc, ch 1, dc) ch 2; rep from * to last 13 ch, (dc, ch 1, dc) in next ch, ch 2, sk 3 ch, (dc, ch 1, dc) in next ch, ch 2, sk 4 ch, (dc, ch 1, dc) in next ch, ch 1, sk 2 ch, dc in last ch.
Row 2 Ch 4 (counts as 1 dc and 1 ch here and throughout), [dc in next dc, dc in next ch-1 sp, dc in next dc, ch 2] across to last 2 dc, dc in next dc, dc in next ch-1 sp, dc in next dc, ch 1, sk 1 ch, dc in next ch.
Row 3 Ch 4, sk next dc, [(dc, ch 1, dc) in next dc, sk next 2 dc and ch-sp, ch 2] across to last 3 dc, (dc, ch 1, dc) in next dc, ch 1, dc in 3rd st of t-ch.
Row 4 Rep row 2.
Row 5 Ch 4, dc2tog, [ch 3, dc2tog] across, ch 1, dc in 3rd st of t-ch.
Row 6 Ch 3 (counts as dc here and throughout), (2 dc, ch 2, 2 dc) in dc2tog, ch 4, sc in next dc2tog, ch 6, sc in next dc2tog, ch 4, *(2 dc, ch 2, 2 dc) in next dc2tog, ch 3, sk next dc2tog, (2 dc, ch 2, 2 dc) in next dc2tog, ch 4, sc in next dc2tog, ch 6, sc in next dc2tog, ch 4; rep from * to last dc2tog, (2 dc, ch 2, 2 dc) in last dc2tog, dc in top st of t-ch.
Row 7 Ch 3, (2 dc, ch 2, 2 dc) in ch-2 sp, ch 1, 9 tr in next ch-6 sp, ch 1, *(2 dc, ch 2, 2 dc) in next ch-2 sp, ch 3, (2 dc, ch 2, 2 dc) in next ch-2 sp, ch 1, 9 tr in next ch-6 sp, ch 1; rep from * to last ch-2 sp, (2 dc, ch 2, 2 dc) in last ch-2 sp, dc in top st of t-ch.

MARLY'S STORY
Marly Bird learned to crochet from her grandmother while at the University of Colorado and was soon stitching during lectures and on track-and-field trips. After college, she went into finance but couldn't ignore the world of crafts: fiber arts, not finance, was for her. She quit her job and started a podcast, *The Yarn Thing*. Marly's designs have appeared in magazines such as *Knit Simple* and *Interweave Crochet*, along with several books, including three especially for plus-size women. Designing for curvy women is near and dear to Marly's heart; she teaches a Craftsy class called Curvy Knits, focusing on fitting techniques. She's lost family members to heart disease, and as a former athlete, she knows the importance of a healthy lifestyle and taking care of her heart. Her design is inspired by Rosemary Chapman, a dear friend who lost her son to heart disease.

MARLY'S TIP
WITH THREE KIDS AND THREE DOGS, Marly has no trouble getting exercise! Having active pets is a great way for you to stay active.

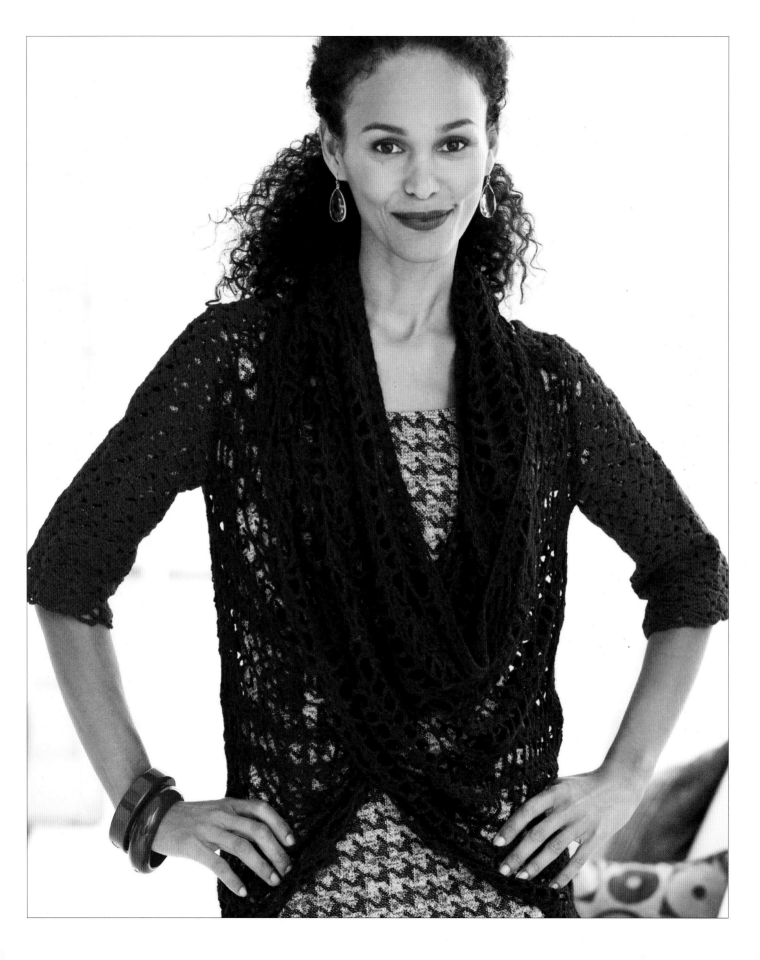

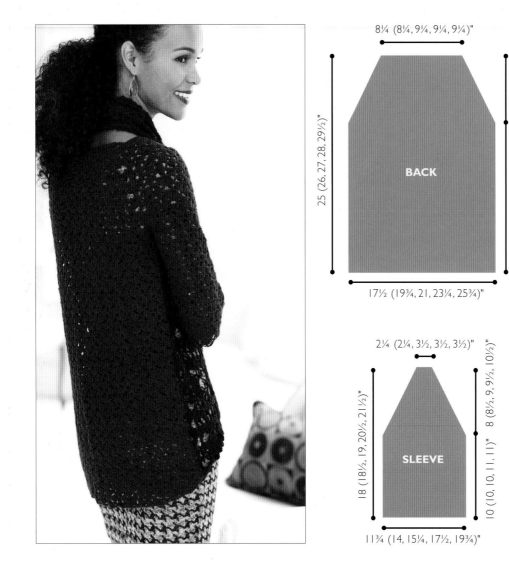

8¼ (8¼, 9¼, 9¼, 9¼)"

BACK

25 (26, 27, 28, 29½)"

8 (8½, 9, 9½, 10½)"

17 (17½, 18, 18½, 19)"

17½ (19¾, 21, 23¼, 25¾)"

2¼ (2¼, 3½, 3½, 3½)"

SLEEVE

8 (8½, 9, 9½, 10½)"

18 (18½, 19, 20½, 21½)"

10 (10, 10, 11, 11)"

11¾ (14, 15¼, 17½, 19¾)"

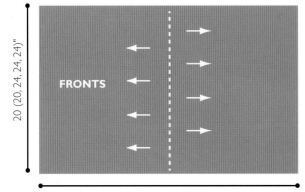

43 (48, 48, 53, 53)"

FRONTS

20 (20, 24, 24, 24)"

86 (96, 96, 106, 106)"

Row 8 Ch 3, (2 dc, ch 2, 2 dc) in ch-2 sp, ch 3, sc in next tr, [ch 4, sk next tr, sc in next tr] 4 times, ch 3, *[(2 dc, ch 2, 2 dc) in next ch-2 sp, ch 3] twice, sc in next tr, [ch 4, sk next tr, sc in next tr] 4 times, ch 3; rep from * to last ch-2 sp, (2 dc, ch 2, 2 dc) in last ch-2 sp, dc in top st of t-ch.

Row 9 Ch 3, (2 dc, ch 2, 2 dc) in ch-2 sp, ch 3, sc in next ch-4 sp, [ch 4, sc in next ch-4 sp] 3 times, ch 3, *(2 dc, ch 2, 2 dc) in next ch-2 sp, ch 3, (2 dc, ch 2, 2 dc) in next ch-2 sp, sc in next ch-4 sp, [ch 4, sc in next ch-4 sp] 3 times, ch 3; rep from * to last ch-2 sp, (2 dc, ch 2, 2 dc) in last ch-2 sp, dc in top st of t-ch.

Row 10 Ch 3, (2 dc, ch 2, 2 dc) in ch-2 sp, [ch 4, sc in next ch-4 sp] 3 times, ch 4, *(2 dc, ch 2, 2 dc) in next ch-2 sp, ch 3, (2 dc, ch 2, 2 dc) in next ch-2 sp, [ch 4, sc in next ch-4 sp] 3 times, ch 4; rep from * to last ch-2 sp, (2 dc, ch 2, 2 dc) in last ch-2 sp, dc in top st of t-ch.

Row 11 Ch 3, (2 dc, ch 2, 2 dc) in ch-2 sp, ch 5, sk next ch-4 sp, sc in next ch-4 sp, ch 4, sc in next ch-4 sp, ch 5, *(2 dc, ch 2, 2 dc) in next ch-2 sp, ch 3, (2 dc, ch 2, 2 dc) in next ch-2 sp, ch 5, sk next ch-4 sp, sc in next ch-4 sp, ch 4, sc in next ch-4 sp, ch 5; rep from * to last ch-2 sp, (2 dc, ch 2, 2 dc) in last ch-2 sp, dc in top st of t-ch.

Row 12 Ch 3, (2 dc, ch 2, 2 dc) in ch-2 sp, ch 8, sc in next ch-4 sp, ch 8, *(2 dc, ch 2, 2 dc) in next ch-2 sp, ch 3, (2 dc, ch 2, 2 dc) in next ch-2 sp, ch 8, sc in next ch-4 sp, ch 8; rep from * to last ch-2 sp, (2 dc, ch 2, 2 dc) in last ch-2 sp, dc in top st of t-ch.

Row 13 Ch 3, (2 dc, ch 2, 2 dc) in ch-2 sp, ch 4, sc in next ch-8 sp, ch 6, sc in next ch-8 sp, ch 4, *(2 dc, ch 2, 2 dc) in next ch-2 sp, ch 3, (2 dc, ch 2, 2 dc) in next ch-2 sp, ch 4, sc in next ch-8 sp, ch 6, sc in next ch-8 sp, ch 4; rep from * to last ch-2 sp, (2 dc, ch 2, 2 dc) in last ch-2 sp, dc in top st of t-ch.
Rep rows 7–13 for pineapple pat, end last rep at row 12.

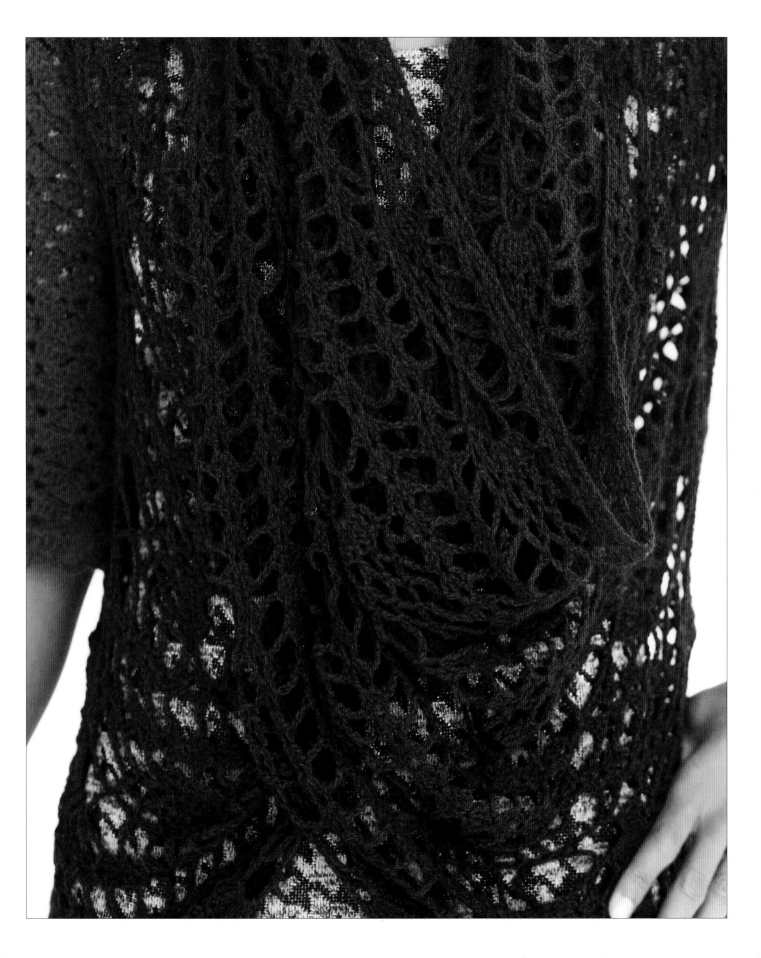

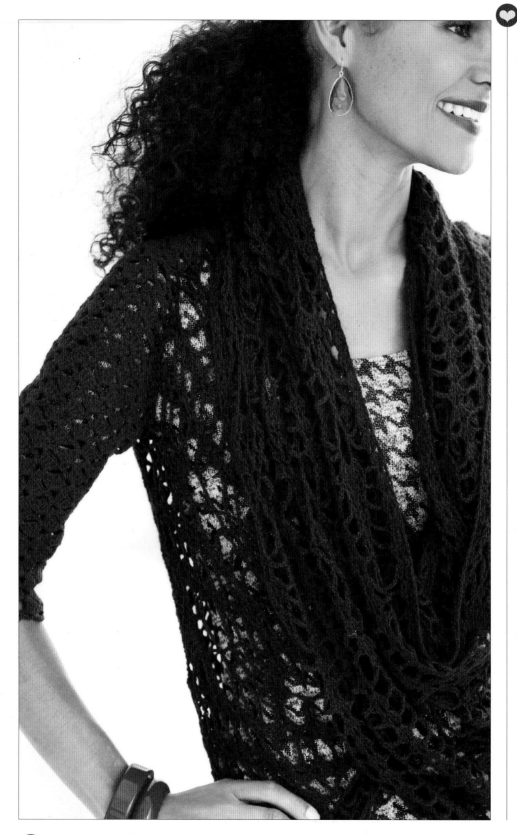

BACK

With A, ch 109 (123, 130, 144, 158). Work 34 (35, 36, 37, 38) rows of asymmetrical pat.

ARMHOLE SHAPING

[Work dec rows 1–3 for 1 (2, 2, 3, 0) times, work 1 row even] 4 (2, 2, 1, 1) times. Work dec rows 1–3 for 0 (1, 1, 3, 7) times, work 0 (0, 1, 0, 0) rows even, fasten off—7 (7, 8, 8, 8) reps.

SLEEVES (MAKE 2)

Using A, ch 74 (88, 95, 109, 123). Work 20 (20, 20, 22, 22) rows of asymmetrical pat.

CAP SHAPING

Work as for back armhole shaping—2 (2, 3, 3, 3) reps.

Block back and sleeves to measurements.
Sew one angled side of each sleeve to each angled side of back to form raglan seams.

FRONT

Using B, ch 108 (108, 129, 129, 129).
*Work rows 1–13 of pineapple pat. Rep rows 7–13 of pat 7 (8, 8, 9, 9) times, ending last rep at row 12.

FINISHING

Pin right side edge of body (side of back plus unsewn raglan edge of sleeve) to final row of front, easing in extra length from body as you pin. Working into ends of rows on body and last row of left front, join pieces as foll:
Ch 2, sc in corner of body, ch 2, sc in 1st ch-sp on front, [ch 2, sc in body, ch 2, sc in next ch-sp of front] across to corners, fasten off.

Working into foundation ch of front, with RS facing, join B with sl st in corner. Ch 4; rep from *. ❤

PINEAPPLE PATTERN

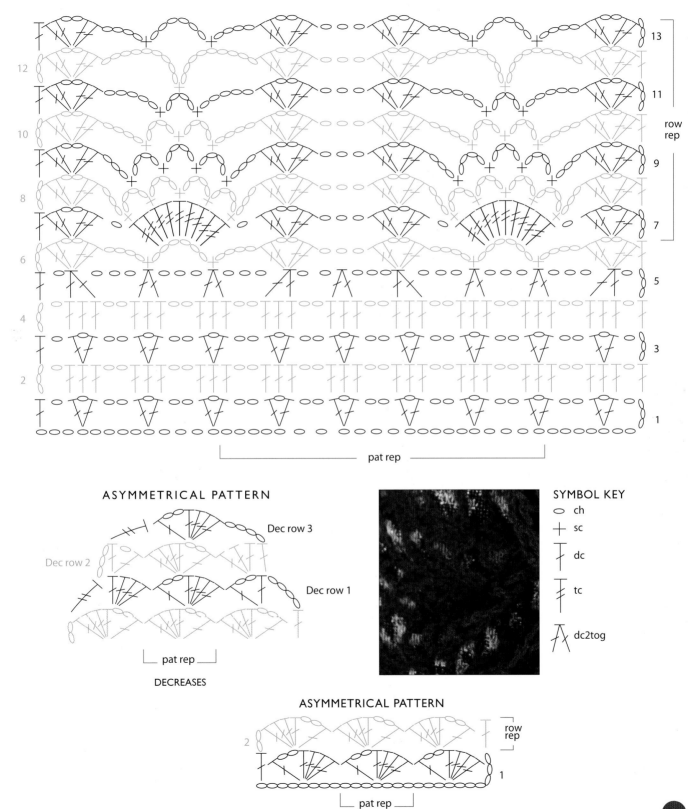

13
12
11
10
9
8
7
6
5
4
3
2
1

row rep

pat rep

ASYMMETRICAL PATTERN

Dec row 3
Dec row 2
Dec row 1

pat rep

DECREASES

SYMBOL KEY

⬭	ch
+	sc
⊤	dc
⊤	tc
⋔	dc2tog

ASYMMETRICAL PATTERN

2
1

row rep

pat rep

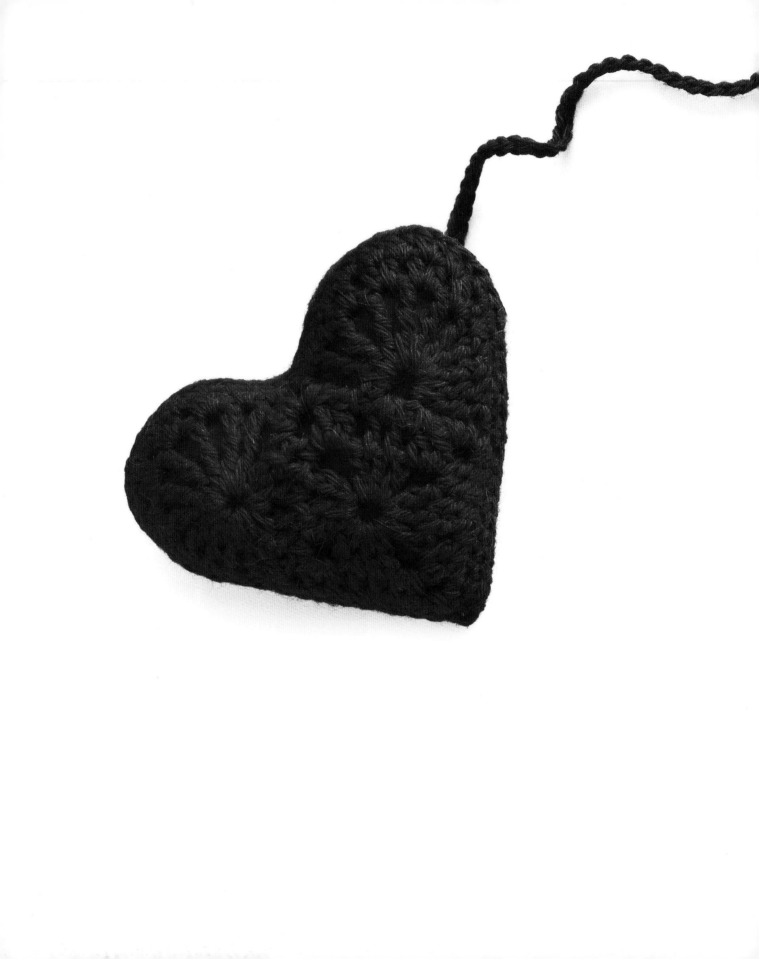

Heart-healthy living

Information, tips, resources, and recipes

Get the facts!

In this book, you've read personal stories from crochet luminaries about their encounters with heart disease and how they look out for their own heart health. Here are some facts that everyone can use to learn more about heart disease and how to fight it.

RED ALERT!

Heart disease is the leading cause of death of women in the United States, but that sobering fact is not common knowledge. Here are a few more eye-opening statistics:

• Both men and women have heart attacks, but more women who have heart attacks die from them.

• Every 90 seconds, a woman in the United States has a heart attack.

• Among all U.S. women who die each year, one in four dies of heart disease.

• In 2004, nearly 60 percent more women died of cardiovascular disease (both heart disease and stroke) than from all cancers combined, and American women are 5 times more likely to die of heart disease than breast cancer.

• More than 10,000 American women younger than 45 have a heart attack every year.

Those are frightening figures, but the good news is that you can take steps to reduce your own risk of heart disease and educate loved ones to protect their hearts.

CHECK IT OUT

One good first step to heart healthiness is to find out how healthy your heart is right now. Here is a list of questions you should ask your doctor or nurse when you go for a physical:

What is my risk for heart disease and stroke?

Which screening or diagnostic tests for heart disease do I need, and when?

What can you do to help me quit smoking?

How much physical activity do I need to help protect my heart and blood vessels?

What is a heart-healthy eating plan for me?

What are my numbers and what do they mean?

☐ Blood pressure

☐ Cholesterol
• Total cholesterol
• LDL ("bad") cholesterol
• HDL ("good") cholesterol
• Triglycerides

☐ Body mass index and waist circumference measurement

☐ Blood sugar level

Once you have a baseline for your heart health, you will be able to track changes and improvements. Your doctor should also be able to tell you about various risk factors that may impact your heart health.

♥ DON'T SMOKE

IF YOU DON'T SMOKE, DON'T EVEN THINK ABOUT STARTING. Smoking carries many health risks beyond heart disease. If you do smoke, make every effort possible to quit. It's the best thing you can do for your health. Talk to your doctor about resources to help you quit, such as nicotine patches.

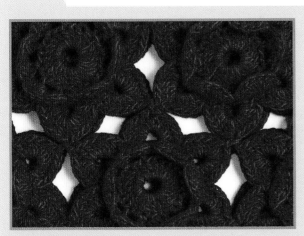

KNOW THE SIGNS

Knowing the signs of a heart attack and what to do when you experience them is one of the most important things you can do for your heart health.

For both women and men, the most common symptom of a heart attack is **pain or discomfort in the center of the chest.** The pain or discomfort can be mild or strong. It can last more than a few minutes, or it can go away and come back.

OTHER COMMON SIGNS OF A HEART ATTACK INCLUDE:

- Pain or discomfort in one or both arms, back, neck, jaw, or stomach
- Shortness of breath (feeling like you can't get enough air), which often occurs before or along with the chest pain or discomfort
- Nausea (feeling sick to your stomach) or vomiting
- Feeling faint or woozy
- Breaking out in a cold sweat
- Swelling in feet, ankles, and legs

Women are more likely than men to have these other common signs of a heart attack, particularly shortness of breath, nausea, or vomiting, and pain in the back, neck, or jaw.

♥ WOMEN ARE ALSO MORE LIKELY TO HAVE LESS COMMON SIGNS OF A HEART ATTACK, INCLUDING:

Heartburn • Loss of appetite • Fatigue or weakness
Coughing • Heart flutters

The signs of a heart attack often occur suddenly, but they can also develop slowly over hours, days, and even weeks before a heart attack occurs. The more heart attack signs that you have, the more likely it is that you are having a heart attack. Also, if you've already had a heart attack, your symptoms may not be the same for another one. Even if you're not sure you're having a heart attack, you should still have it checked out.

If you think you, or someone else, may be having a heart attack, wait no more than a few minutes—five at most—before calling 911.

EAT RIGHT FOR A HEALTHY HEART

Small changes in your diet can make a big difference in your heart health.

BEVERAGES

Take a break from sugary sodas and opt for water with lemon, unsweetened iced tea, or flavored water.

WHOLE GRAINS

Choose whole-grain breads, rice, and noodles, which are packed with important nutrients and are full of fiber to make you feel fuller faster.

SODIUM

Excess sodium has been linked to high blood pressure. Cut back on your sodium by limiting restaurant meals, avoiding processed foods, and using spices other than salt. There are plenty of salt-free spice combinations that you can find in your grocery store. It may take a while for you to get used to the taste, but eventually, you should lose your craving for salt.

POTASSIUM

A potassium-rich diet blunts the harmful effects of sodium on blood pressure. Foods rich in potassium include various fruits and vegetables, especially tomatoes and tomato products, orange juice and grapefruit juice, raisins, dates, and prunes, white potatoes and sweet potatoes, bananas, lettuce, and papayas.

APPETIZERS

Instead of being tempted by fried cheese sticks, opt for fresh fruit, sliced veggies, or salad. Salads should contain fresh greens, other fresh vegetables, and chickpeas. Pass on the high-fat and

high-calorie nonvegetable choices, such as bacon, cheese, and croutons. And what better way to top it off than with lemon juice, vinegar, or a reduced-fat or fat-free dressing?

MAIN DISHES

When cooking at home or eating out, look for some key words on menus or in recipes to know you are making healthier choices. Terms like *skinless, broiled, baked, roasted, poached,* or *lightly sautéed* indicate foods that have been prepared in hearth-healthy ways.

FRUITS AND VEGETABLES

Try to eat at least five servings of fresh fruits and vegetables each day! Choose a variety of produce to maximize the nutritional benefits and keep your plate interesting.

DESSERTS

Although it's probably okay to order that French silk pie for a special occasion, there are plenty of other yummy alternatives to satisfy your sweet tooth. Try fresh fruit, fat-free frozen yogurt, sherbet, or sorbet. If you must indulge, split your dessert with a friend.

♥ DON'T STRESS

Excess stress can raise your blood pressure and increase your risk of a heart attack. Find healthy ways to cope with stress. Lower your stress level by talking to your friends, exercising, or writing in a journal.

Exercise your heart

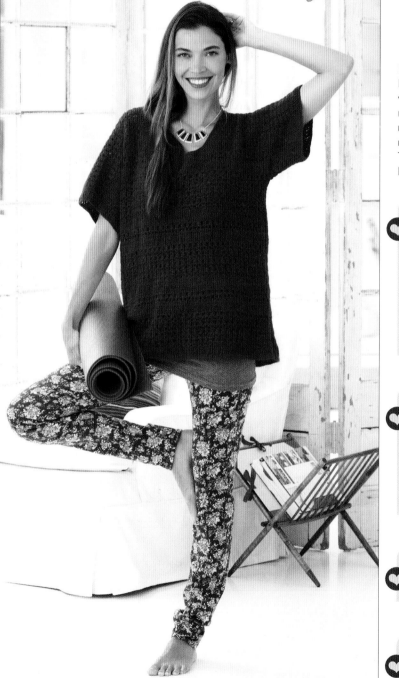

One of the best things you can do for your health is to get up and get active!

Regular exercise can help to maintain a healthy weight, lower blood pressure, and reduce stress—all of which will lower your risk for heart disease. The good news is, you don't have to run a marathon or climb a mountain. The average adult needs only 30 minutes of moderate activity every day to reduce their risk. That's a measly 2% of your day!
Each week aim to get at least:

♥ **2 HOURS AND 30 MINUTES OF MODERATE PHYSICAL ACTIVITY**
During moderate-intensity activities you should notice an increase in your heart rate but still be able to talk comfortably. An example of a moderate-intensity activity is walking on a level surface at a brisk pace (about 3 to 4 miles per hour). Other examples include leisurely bicycling and moderate housework.

OR

♥ **1 HOUR AND 15 MINUTES OF VIGOROUS PHYSICAL ACTIVITY**
If your heart rate increases a lot and you are breathing so hard that it is difficult to carry on a conversation, you are probably doing vigorous-intensity activity. Examples include jogging, bicycling fast or uphill, and singles tennis.

OR

♥ **A COMBINATION OF MODERATE AND VIGOROUS ACTIVITY**

AND

♥ **MUSCLE-STRENGTHENING ACTIVITIES ON TWO OR MORE DAYS**

ADDED BENEFITS

If you need more reasons to start moving, there is strong evidence that regular physical activity can also lower your risk of:

- Stroke
- Type 2 diabetes
- High blood pressure
- Osteoporosis
- Depression
- Unhealthy cholesterol levels
- Colon cancer
- Breast cancer
- Lung cancer

Start slowly in forming exercise habits. Pushing yourself too hard too soon often results in injuries, and those are no fun! If you have concerns or questions about starting an exercise program, talk to your doctor about the best starting place for you.

COVERING ALL THE BASES

In addition to different levels of intensity, there are three types of exercise activity. Make sure to incorporate all three into your workouts on a regular basis.

AEROBIC ACTIVITY

This type most benefits the heart, using large muscle groups and requiring your body to use more oxygen than it normally uses when sitting or resting. Walking, running, and bicycling are good examples.

STRENGTH TRAINING

Strength or resistance training puts excess force on your muscles, making them work harder than normal. Strength training can be structured, with weights or resistance bands, or unstructured, like rock climbing.

FLEXIBILITY ACTIVITIES

Stretching and lengthening your muscles improves joint flexibility, an important factor in injury prevention and maintaining mobility. Practice yoga—or just do some of the simple stretches you did in high school gym class.

MIXING IT UP

Varying your workouts is a great way to ensure that exercise doesn't become boring, and that you're working a variety of muscle groups and getting in all three types of exercise activity.

Some fun workout ideas:
- Take aerobics or weightlifting classes at your gym
- Attend dance classes
- Join a community sports team, such as softball or soccer
- Go for bike rides with friends or family
- Find or create a running group
- Invest in workout DVDs
- Volunteer as a coach or official for local youth sports
- Find a scenic spot to go hiking

MAKING TIME

If you don't schedule time for exercise, it becomes the last priority, something you'll always do tomorrow. Some people have daily rituals like a morning dog walk before sitting down for a cup of coffee, or an after-work run to relieve the day's stress; others change their schedule from day to day.

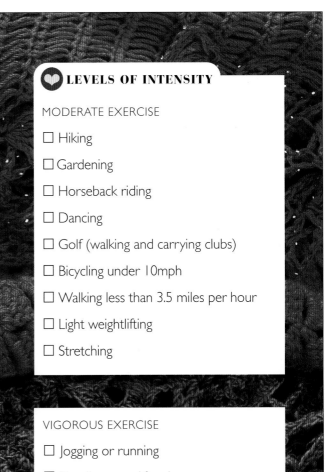

♥ LEVELS OF INTENSITY

MODERATE EXERCISE

- ☐ Hiking
- ☐ Gardening
- ☐ Horseback riding
- ☐ Dancing
- ☐ Golf (walking and carrying clubs)
- ☐ Bicycling under 10mph
- ☐ Walking less than 3.5 miles per hour
- ☐ Light weightlifting
- ☐ Stretching

VIGOROUS EXERCISE

- ☐ Jogging or running
- ☐ Bicycling over 10mph
- ☐ Swimming laps
- ☐ Aerobics and aerobic dancing
- ☐ Walking more than 4.5 miles per hour
- ☐ Heavy yard work, such as chopping wood or shoveling snow
- ☐ Intense weightlifting
- ☐ Singles tennis, racquetball, handball, or squash
- ☐ Team sports such as basketball, soccer, or flag football

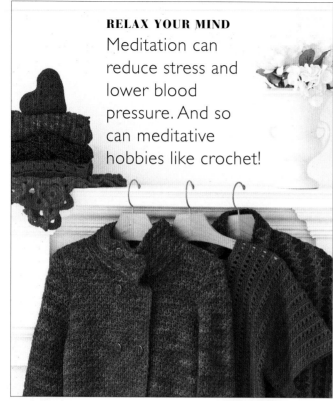

RELAX YOUR MIND

Meditation can reduce stress and lower blood pressure. And so can meditative hobbies like crochet!

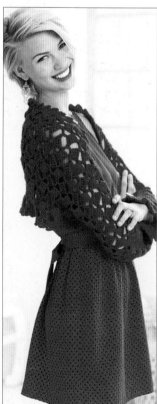

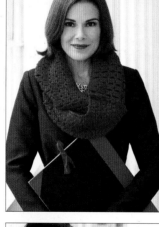

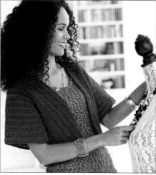

How to keep exercise on your to-do list:
- Make a weekly or monthly workout schedule
- Set aside a specific time each day of the week, whether it's the same time every day or it varies from day to day
- Write down your workouts in your daily planner or enter them in your digital calendar
- Set an alarm or reminder on your cell phone or watch
- Find a workout partner

♥ SAMPLE WEEKLY SCHEDULE

MONDAY	Aerobic; Resistance Training; Flexibility
TUESDAY	Aerobic; Flexibility
WEDNESDAY	Aerobic; Resistance Training; Flexibility
THURSDAY	Aerobic; Flexibility
FRIDAY	Aerobic; Resistance Training; Flexibility
SATURDAY	Aerobic; Flexibility
SUNDAY	Rest OR Aerobic; Flexibility

MAINTAINING MOTIVATION

Let's face it: some days, you just want to relax in front of the TV with a glass of wine—and the last thing you want to do is jump on that treadmill! Here are some incentives to keep your exercise wheels turning:

SET GOALS.
Goals are an excellent way to keep motivated. They can be short-term and simple, like working out 5 days this week or running 5 minutes more than last time; or long-term and complex, like training for a 5K, losing 30 pounds, or learning to tap dance.

LISTEN WHILE YOU WORK OUT.
A favorite podcast, excellent playlists, or a good audio book can make your workout something to look forward to. The time flies by when you're distracted by something fun and engaging.

BUDDY UP.
A date with a workout buddy means you're less likely to stay home. Your buddy relies on you to help her stay motivated, and acts as your personal cheerleader, sharing your goals and wanting you to succeed!

CROCHET ON THE GO!
Squeeze in some quality crochet time during a low-key activity like walking or pedaling on a stationary bike. If walking with a hook isn't up your alley, do 5 push-ups or sit-ups for every 5 minutes you crochet, or spend half an hour exercising for every hour spent crocheting.

REWARD YOURSELF.
Don't forget to pat yourself on the back for a job well done! Give yourself something concrete to look forward to when you accomplish your workout goals. Indulge in a glass of wine, a splurge gift for yourself, or an extra half hour in bed on Sunday. ♥

Read all about it!

Want to learn more? Here are some great resources for finding more information about heart disease and about the steps you can take to make your daily habits more heart healthy.

THE NATIONAL HEART, LUNG, AND BLOOD INSTITUTE AND THE HEART TRUTH®

The Heart Truth is a national awareness and prevention campaign about heart disease in women sponsored by the National Heart, Lung, and Blood Institute (NHLBI), part of the National Institutes of Health of the U.S. Department of Health and Human Services. *The Heart Truth* campaign focuses on the following three areas: professional education, patient education, and public awareness.

CONTACT INFORMATION
www.nhlbi.nih.gov/educational/hearttruth
301-592-8573 • TTY: 240-629-3255
NHLBIinfo@nhlbi.nih.gov

U.S. DEPARTMENT OF HEALTH AND HUMAN SERVICES OFFICE ON WOMEN'S HEALTH

The Office on Women's Health (OWH) offers an award-winning comprehensive website that provide reliable, accurate, commercial-free information on the health of women. They cover more than 800 topics, on issues ranging from adolescent health to reproductive health to healthy aging.

CONTACT INFORMATION
200 Independence Avenue, S.W. , Washington, DC 20201
www.womenshealth.gov
800-994-9662 • TDD: 888-220-5446

ACT IN TIME TO HEART ATTACK SIGNS CAMPAIGN

The National Heart Attack Alert Program is an initiative of the National Heart, Lung, and Blood Institute to alert people to the signs of heart attack.

CONTACT INFORMATION
www.nhlbi.nih.gov/actintime
301-592-8573

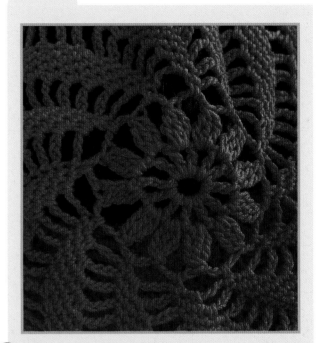

GO TO THE SOURCE
The information in this section was provided by the U.S. Department of Health and Human Services Office on Women's Health, which publishes helpful fact sheets:

HEART DISEASE FACT SHEET
www.womenshealth.gov/publications/our-publications/fact-sheet/heart-disease.cfm

HEART-HEALTHY EATING FACT SHEET
www.womenshealth.gov/publications/our-publications/fact-sheet/heart-healthy-eating.cfm

HEALTH SNAPSHOT: HEART DISEASE
www.womenshealth.gov/publications/our-publications/fact-sheet/health-snapshot/heart-disease-health-snapshot.pdf

HEART ATTACK FACTS: WHAT IS A HEART ATTACK?
www.womenshealth.gov/heartattack/facts.cfm?q=what-is-a-heart-attack

QUESTIONS TO ASK YOUR DOCTOR OR NURSE
www.womenshealth.gov/publications/our-publications/heart-health-stroke-questions.pdf

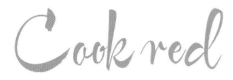
Cook red

You can lighten up your diet without sacrificing flavor. Change a few ingredients and make your favorite dishes more heart-healthy—but just as delicious.

MAIN DISHES

BAKED SALMON DIJON

This salmon entree is easy to make and a delicious treat for family and friends.

INGREDIENTS

1 cup fat-free sour cream

2 teaspoons dried dill

3 tablespoons scallions, finely chopped

2 tablespoons Dijon mustard

2 tablespoons lemon juice

1½ pounds salmon fillet with skin, cut in center

½ teaspoon garlic powder

½ teaspoon black pepper

As needed, fat-free cooking spray

DIRECTIONS

1. Whisk sour cream, dill, onion, mustard, and lemon juice in small bowl to blend.

2. Preheat oven to 400°F. Lightly oil baking sheet with cooking spray.

3. Place salmon, skin side down, on prepared sheet. Sprinkle with garlic powder and pepper. Spread with the sauce.

4. Bake salmon until just opaque in center, about 20 minutes.

Yield: 6 servings

Serving size: 1 piece (4 ounces)

NUTRITION INFORMATION

CALORIES: 196

TOTAL FAT: 7 GRAMS

SATURATED FAT: 2 GRAMS

CHOLESTEROL: 76 MILLIGRAMS

SODIUM: 229 MILLIGRAMS

TOTAL FIBER: LESS THAN 1 GRAM

PROTEIN: 27 GRAMS

CARBOHYDRATES: 5 GRAMS

POTASSIUM: 703 MILLIGRAMS

STIR-FRIED BEEF AND VEGETABLES

This tasty stir-fry dish uses very little oil.

INGREDIENTS

2 tablespoons dry red wine

1 tablespoon soy sauce

½ teaspoon sugar

1½ teaspoons ginger root, peeled, grated

1 pound boneless round steak, fat-trimmed and cut across grain into 1½-inch strips

2 tablespoons vegetable oil

2 medium onions, each cut into 8 wedges

½ pound fresh mushrooms, rinsed, trimmed, and sliced

2 stalks celery, bias-cut into ¼-inch slices

2 small green peppers, cut into thin lengthwise strips

1 cup water chestnuts, drained, sliced

2 tablespoons cornstarch

¼ cup water

DIRECTIONS

1. Prepare marinade by mixing together wine, soy sauce, sugar, and ginger.

2. Marinate meat in mixture while preparing vegetables.

3. Heat 1 tablespoon oil in large skillet or wok. Stir-fry onions and mushrooms for 3 minutes over medium-high heat.

4. Add celery and cook for 1 minute. Add remaining vegetables and cook for 2 minutes or until green pepper is tender but crisp. Transfer vegetables to warm bowl.

5. Add remaining 1 tablespoon oil to skillet. Stir-fry meat in oil for about 2 minutes, or until meat loses its pink color.

6. Blend cornstarch and water. Stir into meat. Cook and stir until thickened.

7. Return vegetables to skillet. Stir gently and serve.

Yield: 6 servings

Serving size: 6 ounces

NUTRITION INFORMATION

CALORIES: 179

TOTAL FAT: 7 GRAMS

SATURATED FAT: 1 GRAM

CHOLESTEROL: 40 MILLIGRAMS

SODIUM: 201 MILLIGRAMS

TOTAL FIBER: 3 GRAMS

PROTEIN: 17 GRAMS

CARBOHYDRATES: 12 GRAMS

POTASSIUM: 552 MILLIGRAMS

BARBECUED CHICKEN

Fall under the spell of this southern-style sweet barbecue sauce.

INGREDIENTS

5 tablespoons (3 ounces) tomato paste

1 teaspoon ketchup

2 teaspoons honey

1 teaspoon molasses

1 teaspoon Worcestershire sauce

4 teaspoons white vinegar

¾ teaspoon cayenne pepper

⅛ teaspoon black pepper

¼ teaspoon onion powder

2 cloves garlic, minced

⅛ teaspoon ginger, grated

1½ pounds chicken (breasts, drumsticks), skinless

DIRECTIONS

1. Combine all ingredients except chicken in saucepan. Simmer for 15 minutes.

2. Wash chicken and pat dry. Place on large platter and brush with ½ of sauce mixture.

3. Cover with plastic wrap and marinate in refrigerator for 1 hour.

4. Place chicken on baking sheet lined with aluminum foil and broil for 10 minutes on each side to seal in juices.

5. Turn down oven to 350°F and add remaining sauce to chicken. Cover chicken with aluminum foil and continue baking for 30 minutes.

Yield: 6 servings

Serving size: ½ breast or 2 small drumsticks

NUTRITION INFORMATION

CALORIES: 176

TOTAL FAT: 4 GRAMS

SATURATED FAT: LESS THAN 1 GRAM

CHOLESTEROL: 81 MILLIGRAMS

SODIUM: 199 MILLIGRAMS

TOTAL FIBER: 1 GRAM

PROTEIN: 27 GRAMS

CARBOHYDRATES: 7 GRAMS

POTASSIUM: 392 MILLIGRAMS

ZUCCHINI LASAGNA

Say "Cheese"! This healthy version of a favorite comfort food will leave you smiling.

INGREDIENTS

½ pound lasagna noodles, cooked
  in unsalted water

¾ cup mozzarella cheese,
  part-skim, grated

1½ cups cottage cheese*, fat free

¼ cups Parmesan cheese, grated

1½ cups zucchini, raw, sliced

2½ cups tomato sauce, no salt added

2 teaspoons basil, dried

2 teaspoons oregano, dried

¼ cup onion, chopped

1 clove garlic

⅛ teaspoon black pepper

DIRECTIONS

1. Preheat oven to 350°F. Lightly spray 9" × 13" baking dish with vegetable oil spray.
2. In small bowl, combine ⅛ cup mozzarella and 1 tablespoon Parmesan cheese. Set aside.
3. In medium bowl, combine remaining mozzarella and Parmesan cheese with all of the cottage cheese. Mix well and set aside.
4. Combine tomato sauce with remaining

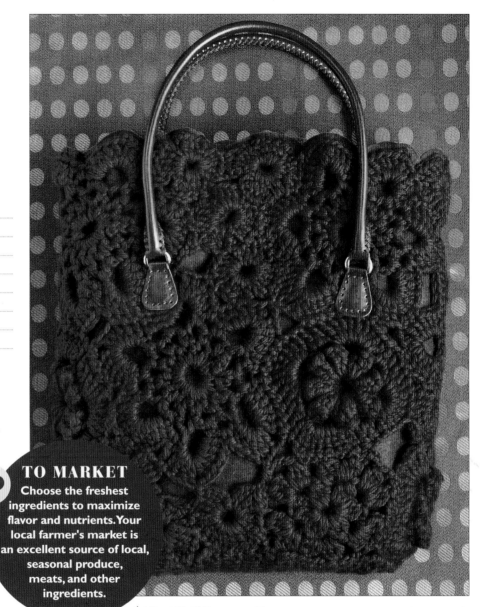

TO MARKET
Choose the freshest ingredients to maximize flavor and nutrients. Your local farmer's market is an excellent source of local, seasonal produce, meats, and other ingredients.

▲ Mixed Motif Tote, page 48

ingredients. Spread thin layer of tomato sauce in bottom of baking dish. Add third of noodles in single layer. Spread half of cottage cheese mixture on top. Add layer of zucchini.
5. Repeat layering.
6. Add thin coating of sauce. Top with noodles, sauce, and reserved cheese mixture. Cover with aluminum foil.
7. Bake for 30–40 minutes. Cool for 10–15 minutes. Cut into 6 portions.

*Use unsalted cottage cheese to reduce the sodium content to 196 mg per serving.

Yield: 6 servings

Serving size: 1 piece

NUTRITION INFORMATION

CALORIES: 276

TOTAL FAT: 5 GRAMS

SATURATED FAT: 2 GRAMS

CHOLESTEROL: 11 MILLIGRAMS

SODIUM: 380 MILLIGRAMS

TOTAL FIBER: 5 GRAMS

PROTEIN: 19 GRAMS

CARBOHYDRATES: 41 GRAMS

POTASSIUM: 561 MILLIGRAM

SIDE DISHES

CLASSIC MACARONI AND CHEESE

Here's a scrumptious, lower-fat version of a favorite dish.

INGREDIENTS

2 cups macaroni

½ cup onions, chopped

½ cup evaporated skim milk

1 medium egg, beaten

¼ teaspoon black pepper

1¼ cup (4 ounces) lowfat sharp cheddar cheese, finely shredded

As needed, nonstick cooking spray

DIRECTIONS

1. Cook macaroni according to directions, but do not add salt to the cooking water. Drain and set aside.
2. Spray casserole dish with nonstick cooking spray. Preheat oven to 350ºF.
3. Lightly spray saucepan with nonstick cooking spray. Add onions and sauté for about 3 minutes.
4. In another bowl, combine macaroni, onions, and rest of ingredients and mix.
5. Transfer mixture into casserole dish.
6. Bake for 25 minutes, or until bubbly. Let stand for 10 minutes before serving.

Yield: 8 servings

Serving size: ½ cup

NUTRITION INFORMATION

CALORIES: 200

TOTAL FAT: 4 GRAMS

SATURATED FAT: 2 GRAMS

CHOLESTEROL: 34 MILLIGRAMS

SODIUM: 120 MILLIGRAMS

TOTAL FIBER: 1 GRAM

PROTEIN: 11 GRAMS

CARBOHYDRATES: 29 GRAMS

POTASSIUM: 119 MILLIGRAMS

SWEET POTATO CUSTARD

Sweet potatoes and bananas combine to make this flavorful, lowfat custard.

INGREDIENTS

1 cup sweet potato, cooked, mashed

½ cup banana (about 2 small), mashed

1 cup evaporated skim milk

2 tablespoons packed brown sugar

2 egg yolks (or ⅓ cup egg substitute), beaten*

½ teaspoon salt

¼ cup raisins

1 tablespoon sugar

1 teaspoon ground cinnamon

As needed, nonstick cooking spray

DIRECTIONS

1. Preheat oven to 325ºF. In medium bowl, stir together sweet potato and banana. Add milk, blending well.
2. Add brown sugar, egg yolks, and salt, mixing thoroughly.
3. Spray 1-quart casserole with nonstick cooking spray. Transfer sweet potato mixture to casserole dish.
4. Combine raisins, sugar, and cinnamon. Sprinkle over top of sweet potato mixture.
5. Bake for 40–45 minutes, or until knife inserted near center comes out clean.
*If using egg substitute, cholesterol will be lower.

Yield: 6 servings

Serving size: ½ cup

NUTRITION INFORMATION

CALORIES: 160

TOTAL FAT: 2 GRAMS

SATURATED FAT: 1 GRAM

CHOLESTEROL: 72 MILLIGRAMS

SODIUM: 255 MILLIGRAMS

TOTAL FIBER: 2 GRAMS

PROTEIN: 5 GRAMS

CARBOHYDRATES: 32 GRAMS

POTASSIUM: 488 MILLIGRAMS

GREEN BEANS SAUTÉ

In this dish, green beans and onions are lightly sautéed in just 1 tablespoon of oil.

INGREDIENTS

1 pound fresh or frozen green beans, cut in 1-inch pieces

1 tablespoon vegetable oil

1 large yellow onion, halved lengthwise, thinly sliced

½ teaspoon salt

⅛ teaspoon black pepper

1 tablespoon fresh parsley, minced

DIRECTIONS

1. If using fresh green beans, cook in boiling water for 10–12 minutes or steam for 2–3 minutes until barely fork tender. Drain well. If using frozen green beans, thaw first.
2. Heat oil in large skillet. Sauté onion until golden.
3. Stir in green beans, salt, and pepper. Heat through.
4. Before serving, toss with parsley.

Yield: 4 servings

Serving Size: ¼ cup

NUTRITION INFORMATION

CALORIES: 64

TOTAL FAT: 4 GRAMS

SATURATED FAT: LESS THAN 1 GRAM

CHOLESTEROL: 0 MILLIGRAMS

SODIUM: 282 MILLIGRAMS

TOTAL FIBER: 3 GRAMS

PROTEIN: 2 GRAMS

CARBOHYDRATES: 8 GRAMS

POTASSIUM: 161 MILLIGRAMS

DESSERTS

APPLE COFFEE CAKE

Apples and raisins keep this cake delectably moist—which means less oil and more heart health.

INGREDIENTS

5 cups tart apples, cored, peeled, chopped

1 cup sugar

1 cup dark raisins

½ cup pecans, chopped

¼ cup vegetable oil

2 teaspoons vanilla

1 egg, beaten

2 cups all-purpose flour, sifted

1 teaspoon baking soda

2 teaspoons ground cinnamon

DIRECTIONS

1. Preheat oven to 350°F. Lightly oil 13" × 9" × 2" pan.
2. In large mixing bowl, combine apples with sugar, raisins, and pecans. Mix well and let stand for 30 minutes.
3. Stir in oil, vanilla, and egg.
4. Sift together flour, soda, and cinnamon, and stir into apple mixture about ⅓ at a time—just enough to moisten dry ingredients.
5. Turn batter into pan. Bake for 35–40 minutes. Cool cake slightly before serving.

Yield: 20 servings

Serving size: 3½-inch × 2½-inch piece

NUTRITION INFORMATION

CALORIES: 196

TOTAL FAT: 8 GRAMS

SATURATED FAT: 1 GRAM

CHOLESTEROL: 11 MILLIGRAMS

SODIUM: 67 MILLIGRAMS

TOTAL FIBER: 2 GRAMS

PROTEIN: 3 GRAMS

CARBOHYDRATES: 31 GRAMS

POTASSIUM: 136 MILLIGRAMS

1-2-3 PEACH COBBLER

Try this healthier, mouth-watering take on a classic.

INGREDIENTS

½ teaspoon ground cinnamon

1 tablespoon vanilla extract

2 tablespoons cornstarch

1 cup peach nectar

¼ cup pineapple or peach juice (can use juice from canned peaches)

2 cans (16 ounces each) peaches, packed in juice, drained (or 1¾ pound fresh), sliced

1 tablespoon tub margarine

1 cup dry pancake mix

⅔ cup all-purpose flour

½ cup sugar

⅔ cup evaporated skim milk

½ teaspoon nutmeg

1 tablespoon brown sugar

As needed, nonstick cooking spray

DIRECTIONS

1. Combine cinnamon, vanilla, cornstarch, peach nectar, and pineapple or peach juice in saucepan over medium heat. Stir constantly until mixture thickens and bubbles.
2. Add sliced peaches to mixture. Reduce heat and simmer for 5–10 minutes.
3. In another saucepan, melt margarine and set aside.
4. Lightly spray 8-inch square glass dish with cooking spray. Pour in peach mixture.
5. In another bowl, combine pancake mix, flour, sugar, and melted margarine. Stir in milk. Quickly spoon this mixture over peach mixture.
6. Combine nutmeg and brown sugar. Sprinkle mixture on top of batter.
7. Bake at 400°F for 15–20 minutes, or until golden brown. Cool and cut into 8 squares.

Yield: 8 servings

Serving size: 1 square

NUTRITION INFORMATION

CALORIES: 271

TOTAL FAT: 4 GRAMS

SATURATED FAT: LESS THAN 1 GRAM

CHOLESTEROL: LESS THAN 1 MILLIGRAM

SODIUM: 263 MILLIGRAMS

TOTAL FIBER: 2 GRAMS

PROTEIN: 4 GRAMS

CARBOHYDRATES: 54 GRAMS

POTASSIUM: 284 MILLIGRAMS

♥ KEEP COOKING!

These fabulous recipes were provided by the National Heart, Lung, and Blood Institute. For more delicious, heart-healthy recipes, go to: www.nhlbi.nih.gov/health/public/heart/other/ktb_recipebk/ktb_recipebk.pdf

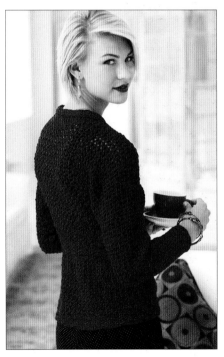

▲ Peplum Jacket, page 16

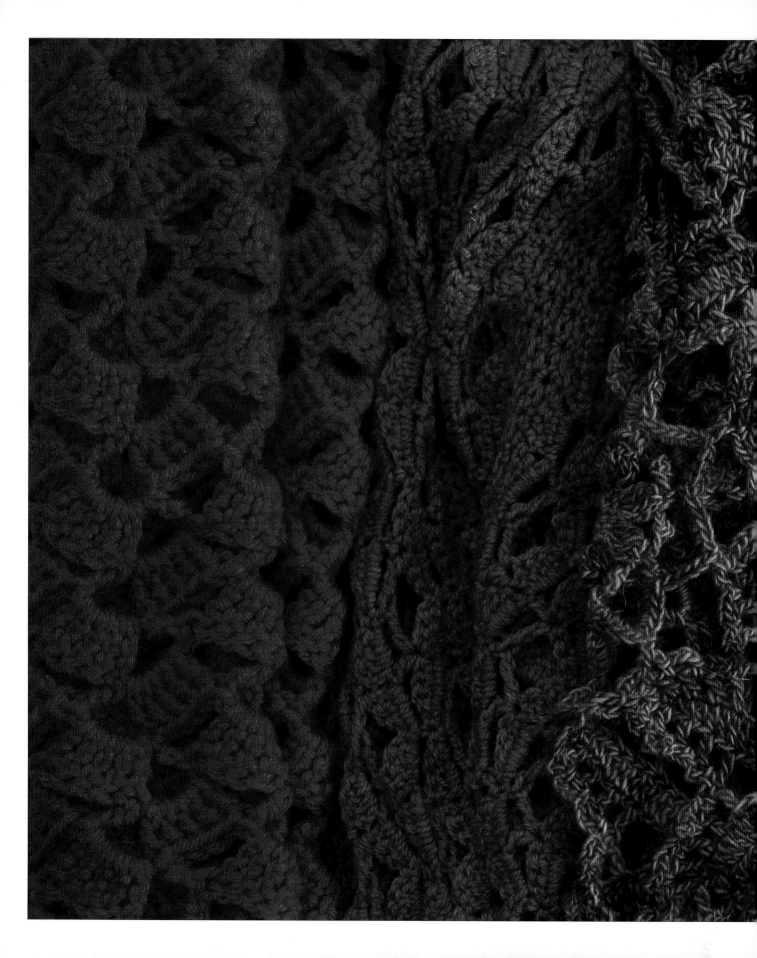

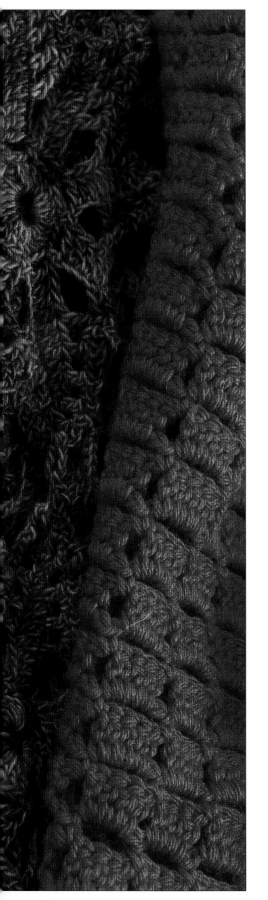

crochet know-how

♥ ABBREVIATIONS

approx approximately

beg begin; beginning; begins

BP dc back post double crochet

ch chain; chains

cl cluster

cont continue; continuing

dc double crochet

dec decrease; decreasing

dtr double treble crochet

foll follow(s)(ing)

FP dc front post double crochet

grp(s) group(s)

hdc half double crochet

inc increase; increasing

lp(s) loop(s)

pat(s) pattern(s)

RS right side

rem remain; remains; remaining

rep repeat

reverse sc reverse single crochet (aka crab stitch)

rnd(s) round(s)

sc single crochet

sc2tog single crochet two together

sk skip

sl slip; slipping

sl st slip stitch

sp(s) space(s)

st(s) stitch(es)

tbl through back loop

t-ch turning chain

tfl through front loop

tog together

tr treble crochet

trtr triple treble crochet

WS wrong side

work even continue in pattern without increasing or decreasing

yo yarn over hook

( ) work instructions contained inside the parentheses into the stitch indicated

[ ] rep instructions within brackets as many times as directed

* rep instructions following an asterisk as many times as indicated

♥ CROCHET HOOKS

U.S.	METRIC
B/1	**2.25mm**
C/2	2.75mm
D/3	**3.25mm**
E/4	3.5mm
F/5	**3.75mm**
G/6	4mm
7	**4.5mm**
H/8	5mm
I/9	**5.5mm**
J/10	6mm
K/10½	**6.5mm**
L/11	8mm
M/13	**9mm**
N/15	10mm

SKILL LEVELS

■□□□
1. BEGINNER
Ideal first project.

■■□□
2. EASY
Basic stitches, minimal shaping, and simple finishing.

■■■□
3. INTERMEDIATE
For crocheters with some experience. More intricate stitches, shaping, and finishing.

■■■■
4. EXPERIENCED
For crocheters able to work patterns with complicated shaping and finishing.

♥ **METRIC CONVERSIONS**
To convert measurements from inches to centimeters, simply multiply by 2.54.

STANDARD YARN WEIGHT SYSTEM

Categories of yarn, gauge ranges, and recommended needle and hook sizes

Yarn Weight Symbol & Category Names	0 Lace	1 Super Fine	2 Fine	3 Light	4 Medium	5 Bulky	6 Super Bulky
Type of Yarns in Category	Fingering 10 count crochet thread	Sock, Fingering, Baby	Sport, Baby	DK, Light Worsted	Worsted, Afghan, Aran	Chunky, Craft, Rug	Bulky, Roving
Knit Gauge Range* in Stockinette Stitch to 4 inches	33 –40** sts	27–32 sts	23–26 sts	21–24 sts	16–20 sts	12–15 sts	6–11 sts
Recommended Needle in Metric Size Range	1.5–2.25 mm	2.25–3.25 mm	3.25–3.75 mm	3.75–4.5 mm	4.5–5.5 mm	5.5–8 mm	8 mm and larger
Recommended Needle U.S. Size Range	000 to 1	1 to 3	3 to 5	5 to 7	7 to 9	9 to 11	11 and larger
Crochet Gauge* Ranges in Single Crochet to 4 inch	32-42 double crochets**	21–32 sts	16–20 sts	12–17 sts	11–14 sts	8–11 sts	5–9 sts
Recommended Hook in Metric Size Range	Steel*** 1.6–1.4mm Regular hook 2.25 mm	2.25–3.5 mm	3.5–4.5 mm	4.5–5.5 mm	5.5–6.5 mm	6.5–9 mm	9 mm and larger
Recommended Hook U.S. Size Range	Steel*** 6, 7, 8 Regular hook B–1	B–1 to E–4	E–4 to 7	7 to I–9	I–9 to K–10½	K–10½ to M–13	M–13 and larger

* Guidelines only: The above reflect the most commonly used gauges and needle or hook sizes for specific yarn categories.

** Lace weight yarns are usually knitted or crocheted on larger needles and hooks to create lacy, openwork patterns. Accordingly, a gauge range is difficult to determine. Always follow the gauge stated in your pattern.

*** Steel crochet hooks are sized differently from regular hooks—the higher the number, the smaller the hook, which is the reverse of regular hook sizing.

CONVERSION CHART

U.S. Term	U.K./AUS Term
sl st (slip stitch)	sc (single crochet)
sc (single crochet)	dc (double crochet)
hdc (half double crochet)	htr (half treble crochet)
dc (double crochet)	tr (treble crochet)
tr (treble crochet)	dtr (double treble crochet)
dtr (double treble crochet)	trip tr or trtr (triple treble crochet)
trtr (triple treble crochet)	qtr (quadruple treble crochet)
rev sc (reverse single crochet)	rev dc (reverse double crochet)
yo (yarn over)	yoh (yarn over hook)

♥ TOOLS OF THE TRADE

Simulated bone hook (plastic)

Standard aluminum hook

Large plastic hook for bulky yarn

Extra-large hook for super-bulky yarn

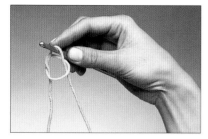

SLIPKNOT

Make a loop, placing one end of the yarn centered underneath the loop. Insert the hook under the center strand and pull it up into a loop on the hook. Pull both yarn ends to tighten the knot on the hook.

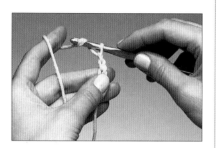

FOUNDATION CHAIN

1. Place the head of the hook under the long end of the yarn. The yarn should lie over the hook from back to front. This is called "yarn over."

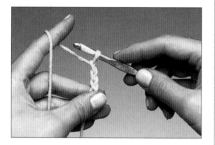

2. Pull the yarn-over through the loop already on the hook—one chain has been completed.

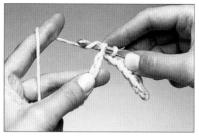

SINGLE CROCHET

1. Make a foundation chain of desired length. Insert the hook under 2 loops of the next chain stitch and yarn over. (On a foundation row, start in the second chain from the hook.)

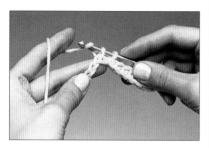

2. Draw the yarn-over through the chain, then yarn over once again. (There are now 2 loops on the hook plus the new yarn-over.)

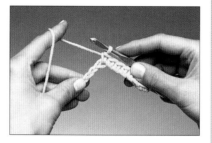

3. Draw the new yarn-over through the 2 loops on the hook—one single crochet completed.

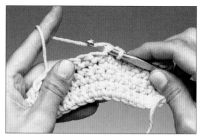

SLIP STITCH

1. Insert the hook under both of the top 2 loops of the next stitch and yarn over.

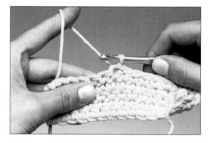

2. Draw the yarn-over through the stitch and the loop on the hook in one motion.

GET A GRIP!

Remember when you were first learning how to write? In the beginning the motions felt awkward. With repetition, however, they became second nature. Learning to crochet is much the same. Your dominant hand holds the hook—hand on top, as shown in these photos, or from below, like a pencil.

With your other hand, you "feed" the yarn and control the tension. One way is by holding the yarn away from the work with the index finger, as shown in these photos. Another way is to hold the index finger closer to the work, with the yarn going over the index finger and under the remaining fingers. Experiment to find the most comfortable technique for you.

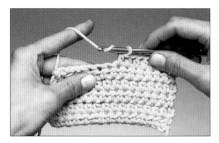

HALF DOUBLE CROCHET
1. To begin a half double crochet stitch, yarn over.

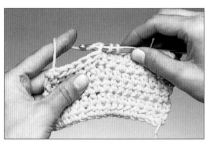

2. Insert hook under the 2 top loops of the next stitch and yarn over.

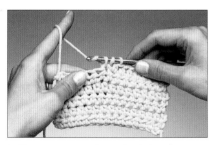

3. Draw yarn-over through stitch; yarn over again.

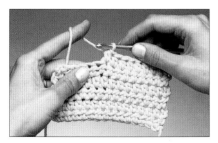

4. Draw yarn-over through all 3 loops on hook—one half double crochet completed.

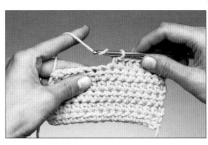

DOUBLE CROCHET
1. To begin a double crochet stitch, yarn over.

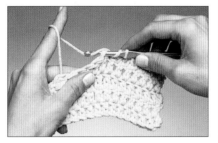

2. Insert hook under the 2 top loops of the next stitch and yarn over once again.

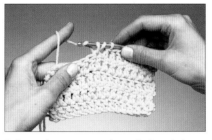

3. Draw the yarn-over through the stitch— 3 loops are on hook; yarn over once again.

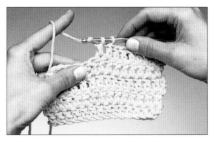

4. Draw yarn-over through first 2 loops; yarn over once again. Draw yarn-over through last 2 loops on hook to complete double crochet.

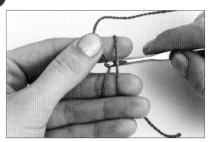

ADJUSTABLE RING
1. To begin the adjustable ring, wrap the yarn loosely around two fingers, the loose tail near your fingertips and the working yarn to the inside.

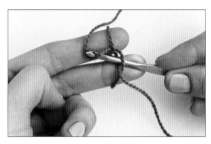

2. With the crochet hook, bring the working strand under the outside strand, then draw a loop through, as shown.

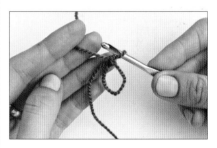

3. Draw through another loop to complete the single crochet. When all the stitches for the beginning of the pattern have been worked into the ring, close the ring by pulling the loose tail.

♥ **BONUS PATTERN BY KRISTIN NICHOLAS**

Heart Sachet

Fill this sweet fabric-lined heart with soothing potpourri scents, as a reminder to stay relaxed and heart-healthy!

◼◼◻◻

MEASUREMENTS
WIDTH AT WIDEST POINT
5½"/14cm
HEIGHT AT CENTER
4"/10cm

MATERIALS
• 1 1¾oz/50g ball (each approx 93yd/85m) of Classic Elite Yarns *Color By Kristin* (wool/mohair/alpaca) in #3258 geranium (④)
• Size G/6 (4mm) crochet hook
• ¼yd/1.25m red quilting-weight cotton for lining
• Small amount of polyfill stuffing
• Potpourri (optional)
• Sewing needle and thread

BACK
RIGHT LOBE
Ch 4, join with sl st to form ring.
Next row Ch 4, 5 tr in ring, 6 dtr in ring. Fasten off.

LEFT LOBE
Ch 4, join with sl st to form ring.
Next row Ch 5, 5 dtr in ring, 6 tr in ring. Fasten off.

LOWER PORTION
Ch 4, join with sl st to form ring.
Rnd 1 Ch 3, 2 dc in ring, [ch 2 (for corner) 3 dc in ring] 3 times, ch 3, join with sl st to top of beg-ch.
Rnd 2 Ch 3, [1 dc in space between next 2 dc] twice, *2 dc in ch-2 sp, ch 2, 2 dc in ch-2 sp, [1 dc in space between next 2

dc] twice; rep from * twice more, 2 dc in ch-2 sp, ch 2, 1 dc in ch-2 sp, join with sl st to top of beg-ch. Fasten off—6 dc across each side of square.
With dtrs of each lobe meeting at center top corner, sew right and left lobes to 2 sides of square using an overhand stitch.

BORDER
Rnd 1 Join yarn with sl st to bottom point of square, ch 1, work 2 sc in ch-2 sp, 5 sc evenly along side of square; working in right lobe, work 2 sc in ch-2sp, [1 sc in space between next 2 tr] 5 times, [2 hdc in space between next 2 dtr] 4 times, [1 sc between next 2 dtr] twice to center of heart; working in left lobe, [1 sc between next 2 dtr] twice, [2 hdc in space between next 2 dtr] 4 times, [1 sc in space between next 2 tr] 5 times, 5 sc along side of square, 2 sc in ch-sp, ch 2. Join with sl st to beg ch-1.
Next rnd Ch 1, sc in sp between each sc, then 2 hdc between each hdc—16 hdc on each side. Ch 2 and fasten off, leaving 20"/50cm tail for sewing together.

FRONT
Work as for back.

FINISHING
INNER HEART
Using the crochet heart as a template, cut 2 pieces of the cotton fabric. With right sides together, sewing needle and thread, sew fabric hearts tog leaving a ¼"/.5cm seam allowance and leaving 2"/5cm open for stuffing. Turn right side out and press. Stuff with polyfill and/or potpourri. Sew closed.

OUTER HEART
Place crochet hearts with wrong sides tog. With tapestry needle and yarn, whipstitch around, leaving opening for inner heart. Place inner heart into crochet heart and sew closed.♥

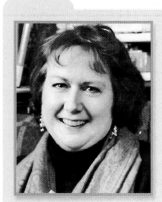

KRISTIN'S STORY
While her hobbies range from interior decorating to painting, Kristin Nicholas has always wanted to be a fashion designer. She learned to crochet as a girl from her grandmother, and her love of color and the fiber arts led to two degrees in textiles and clothing, followed by a sixteen-year stint as creative director of Classic Elite Yarns. Kristin finds inspiration in the world around her—from art books and flowers to ethnic textiles. She and her husband, their daughter, three border collies, one Great Pyrenees, and several cats all live on an idyllic farm in western Massachusetts, where they raise sheep and chickens—which means Kristin gets plenty of exercise to keep her heart in shape. But a healthy diet is just as important: she and her husband sell their high-quality, grass-fed lamb locally, and Kristin develops healthy recipes featuring the nutritious, natural meat and cooks vitamin-rich stock made from the lamb bones.

♥ **KRISTIN'S TIP**
EAT NATURAL, GRASS-FED MEATS. Kristin raises her lambs without antibiotics or hormones and feeds them only fresh grass and hay.

❤ YARN RESOURCES

To locate retailers, contact the manufacturers listed below.

ARTYARNS
39 Westmoreland Avenue
White Plains, NY 10606
www.artyarns.com

BERNAT
320 Livingstone Avenue South
Box 40
Listowel, ON N4W 3H3
Canada
www.bernat.com

BERROCCO, INC.
1 Tupperware Drive, Suite 4
North Smithfield, RI 02896-6815
www.berroco.com

BIJOU BASIN RANCH
P.O. Box 154
Elbert, CO 80106
bijoubasinranch.com

BLUE SKY ALPACAS, INC.
P.O. Box 88
Cedar, MN 55011
blueskyalpacas.com

CASCADE YARNS
1224 Andover Park East
Tukwila, WA 98188
www.cascadeyarns.com

CLASSIC ELITE YARNS
122 Western Avenue
Lowell, MA 01851
www.classiceliteyarns.com

COATS & CLARK
Consumer Services
P.O. Box 12229
Greenville, SC 29612-0229
www.coatsandclark.com

DEBBIE BLISS
Distributed by Knitting Fever
www.debbieblissonline.com

DEBORAH NORVILLE
COLLECTION
Distributed by Premier Yarns

DREW EMBORSKY
www.drewemborsky.com

ERIKA KNIGHT
10 Bush Mews
Arundel Road
Brighton BN2 5TE
United Kingdom
www.erikaknight.co.uk

FYBERSPATES
Unit 1 + 6 Oxleaze farm
workshops
Broughton Poggs
Filkins
Lechlade
Glos, GL7 3RB
United Kingdom
www.fyberspates.co.uk

HAMILTON YARNS
1468 Keys Crossing Drive
Atlanta, GA 30319
www.hamiltonyarns.com

HANDMAIDEN FINE YARN
handmaiden.ca

HIKOO
Distributed by
Skacel Collection, Inc.

KNITTING FEVER (KFI)
P.O. Box 336
315 Bayview Avenue
Amityville, NY 11701
www.knittingfever.com

LION BRAND YARN CO.
34 West 15th Street
New York, NY 10011
www.lionbrand.com

LORNA'S LACES
4229 North Honore Street
Chicago, IL 60613
www.lornaslaces.net

MADELINETOSH
7515 Benbrook Pkwy
Benbrook, TX 76126
madelinetosh.com

MALABRIGO YARN
www.malabrigoyarn.com

MUENCH YARNS, INC.
1323 Scott Street
Petaluma, CA 94954-1135
www.myyarn.com

NORO
Distributed by Knitting Fever

PREMIER YARNS
284 Ann Street
Concord, NC 28025
sales@premieryarns.com

RED HEART LTD.
A Coats & Clark Brand
www.redheart.com

ROWAN
Distributed by
Westminster Fibers

SHIBUI KNITS, LLC
1500 NW 18th, Suite 110
Portland, OR 97209
info@shibuiknits.com

SKACEL COLLECTION, INC.
www.skacelknitting.com

STONEHEDGE FIBER MILL
2246 Pesek Road
East Jordan, MI 49727
www.stonehedgefibermill.com

SWANS ISLAND YARNS
231 Atlantic Highway
(Route 1)
Northport, ME 04849
www.swansislandcompany.com

SWEETGEORGIA YARNS INC.
110-408 East Kent Avenue
Vancouver, BC V5X 2X7
Canada
www.sweetgeorgiayarns.com

TAHKI•STACY CHARLES, INC.
70-30 80th Street, Building 36
Ridgewood, NY 11385
www.tahkistacycharles.com

WESTMINSTER FIBERS
165 Ledge Street
Nashua, NH 03060
www.westminsterfibers.com

INDEX

❤ CREDITS

PORTRAITS OF DESIGNERS
p. 16: Patrick Moos
p. 22: Chris Vaccaro
p. 24: Michael Luppino
p. 28: Alan B. Silverman
p. 31: Jarrod Sumpter
p. 34: Mel White
p. 36: Timothy Sanders White
p. 39: Mark Miller
p. 42: Harrison Stone
p. 45: Gary Hickman
p. 48: Alastair Muir
p. 51: Sebastian Voth
p. 57: Barry Alsop
p. 60: Heather Weston
p. 64: Richard Burns
p. 66: Elliot Schreier
p. 69: Sheila Rock
p. 73: R. A. Sullivan
p. 76: Rose Callahan
p. 81: Dora Ohrenstein
p. 85: Selma Moss-Ward
p. 89: Mark Chachula
p. 92: Keith Brofsky
p. 94: Alex Kaplan
p. 97: Aaron Miller
p. 102: Grant Delin
p. 106: Richard Hanley
p. 109: Jack Deutsch
p. 112: Jim Forni
p. 116: Karen Julliano
p. 140: Jack Deutsch

♥ ACKNOWLEDGMENTS

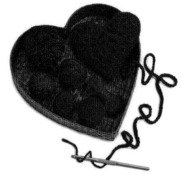

Crochet Red is my third book to be published, and if I have learned anything, it would be that authoring books does not get easier the more you publish. Each volume is a unique journey with its own challenges and rewards, and I am extremely grateful to have had the support of so many incredible individuals throughout the course of creating the Stitch Red books. *Knit Red*, *Sew Red*, and now *Crochet Red* have all given me the opportunity to collaborate with talented designers, exceptional yarn companies, and the wonderful staff at Sixth&Spring Books; I am honored to have had the pleasure of working with all of you to create something so meaningful and close to my heart.

I offer an extra-special thank you to the following individuals who went above and beyond and were integral in making *Crochet Red* the book you are holding in your hands, a book we are all so proud of.

Leanne Spinazola, for jumping in at the last minute without hesitation. Thank you for keeping so many details organized, for researching, writing, and editing (Heather Boyd, too!), for turning my random thoughts into intelligible sentences . . . and for simply being LeAwesome.

Rose Callahan, for being the best photographer in the world. Your pictures bring the Stitch Red books to life, and it is because of you and super-talented stylist Khaliah Jones that they are so successful.

Kaity Ocean, for working tirelessly to make this Stitch Red campaign everything it is today. You have poured your heart and soul (and a few glasses of red wine!) into this project . . . and it shows!

I would like to reiterate a most sincere thank you to all the designers and yarn companies who so selflessly dedicated their time and energy to this project. Without your enthusiasm, creativity, and passion, *Crochet Red* would not have become an exceptional resource, and I am truly grateful to have you as part of this book. If we can get just one person to pay better attention to heart health as a result of our efforts, we have succeeded. Together.

Last but certainly not least, I want to give a heartfelt thanks to the people in my day-to-day life who cheered me on through this endeavor: my family and friends at Jimmy Beans Wool. Both the staff members and the customers of the Biggest Little Yarn Shop in Reno are a constant source of inspiration, technical expertise, moral support, and just plain fun. Thank you all for being the bedrock underneath this mountain we're building together. ♥